Reviews

"Spiritual seekers find truths in many places. For Jews in particular, whose souls are especially hungry, this presents a challenge and an opportunity: how to reconcile various paths with the rich tradition of our Jewish heritage. In Wrestling with Yoga, Shelly Dembe has done a great service in sharing her unique story, revealing the struggle of a Jewish soul learning to navigate between spiritual disciplines and finding peace as a Jew. Her extraordinary mosaic uncovers deeper truths in Judaism."
Rabbi Simon Jacobson, "Toward A Meaningful Life"

"A beautiful and honest exploration of her own practice of yoga and Judaism. A portrait of an examined life where curiosity is an essential value. Crisp and clear, inviting readers to walk with her toward a more spiritually fulfilling and balanced life."
Susan Berrin, Editor-in-Chief
Sh'ma: A Journal of Jewish Responsibility

"Her clarity and humility are a testament to the mindfulness and courageous search for truth that underscore her life and the book her journey has produced. She outlines her battle and her awakenings and inspires each of us to wrestle with our own blind spots and move into the light."
Shimona Tzukernik, The Kabbalah Coach

"Shelly Dembe's sincere and honest effort to recontextualize yoga practice in an authentic Jewish spiritual context documents her initial reservations and gradual acceptance of Jewish spirituality. In so doing, she portrays a deep and multi-layered spirituality and presents the basic rituals and prayers of the day, week and year as tools for the mindful, conscious lifestyle."
Rabbi Pinchas Giller, Chair, Jewish Studies, American Jewish University

"A clearly told reflection on how the practice of yoga can inspire us to see under the surface of our religious traditions and lead a life of deep and sacred connection."
Edi Pasalis, Associate Director, Institute for Extraordinary Living
Kripalu Center for Yoga & Health

More Reviews...

"Engrossing, delightful memoir of an unusual journey to Jewish tradition through the melding of two cultures."
Rochelle L. Millen, PhD, Professor of Religion
Wittenberg University

"A warm, funny, thoughtful voice tackling an important subject. She lives her life as if what she does matters in every moment, testing her experiences against her faith, and shares the struggle with you. This book will resonate not just with Jews grappling with being true to their beliefs but with everyone tempted to dip a toe into Eastern practices like yoga or Buddhist meditation without compromising the faith that sustains them."
Linda Oshins, Co-Founder, Yoga on High

"Yoga has been of great interest to many members of the Jewish community. Yet there are numerous elements of traditional yoga that contradict Judaism, especially its most urgent demand that there be no connection to any perceived or imagined power in any way whatsoever other than to the one G-d as defined by the Torah.
Shelly has done an excellent job in this book of peeling away those elements of yoga that contradict Judaism while retaining those concepts that are neutral and hence of utility to enhance physical, emotional well being—matters of great importance to Judaism. She also explores those moral and ethical ideas within yoga that do not seem to contradict Judaism, or invoke any other higher power or authority.
This is not a general endorsement of any form of involvement in any type of yoga: the question remains open as to whether an individual ought to practice yoga even in this modified form, an individuated question that should be addressed by each individual to the person who is their personal source of Halachic and general Judaic guidance."
Rabbi Shlomo Yaffe, Institute for Judaic Knowledge

ב"ה

Dear Yehudis Chana,

Wishing you brachas
for joy, exuberant health,
love & growth in Torah.
So nice to know you!

Shelly Dembe

© 2013 Shelly Dembe
Printed in the United States of America
ISBN 978-0-9829841-2-3

Published by HealthSprings Media
www.HealthSpringsMedia.com
Dallas, TX

1.2

Publisher's Cataloging-In-Publication Data
Dembe, Shelly.
    Wrestling with yoga : journey of a Jewish soul / Shelly Dembe.
        p. : ill. ; cm.
    Includes bibliographical references and index.
    ISBN: 978-0-9829841-2-3

    1. Dembe, Shelly--Religion. 2. Spiritual life--Judaism. 3. Yoga--Religious aspects. 4. Hinduism--Relations--Judaism. 5. Judaism--Relations--Hinduism. I. Title.
BM538.Y64 D46 2013
296.39   2013949471

To my parents,
whose unconditional love and belief
in my abilities carry me through life.
You have filled my well with
curiosity, abundance and joy.

Acknowledgements

Many wise, insightful and generous people shared their experiences, knowledge and support during my personal spiritual journey, and many contributed to the book which has resulted. My heartfelt appreciation is extended to:

All of my students across the country. It is because of you that I wrote this book. I am so grateful for the blessing of learning through teaching all of you. Your questions propel me further on the path of truth. And to those who come to dance with me...thank you for sharing my joy!

My yoga teachers for laying the foundation for a lifelong practice on and off the mat: Linda Chappell, Judith Baker, Wendy Dion, Megha Nancy Buttenheim and to my teachers at Yoga on High, Columbus, Ohio:

Martha Marcum, Marcia Miller, and especially Linda Oshins for your continued mentoring, friendship and inspiration.

All of the *shluchim* who took a chance and brought me in to share dance and halachically safe yoga with your community. The curiosity of the women in your circle coaxed me into researching the material for this book.

To my Columbus, Ohio community for providing a friendly, accessible and non-judgmental place to come home to.

Rabbi Simon Jacobson for his insight, clarity and assurance that the writing of this book made sense.

Rabbi Levi Andrusier, Rabbi Avi Ben Moshe, Rabbi Chaim Capland, Chani Capland, Sara Deitsch, Rabbi William Goldberg, Rabbi Yosef Gopin, Rabbi Aryeh Kaltmann, Esther Kaltmann and Rabbi Shlomo Yaffe for answering my many questions and teaching me the beauty of *Chassidus*.

Rabbi Chaim Yosef Ackerman, Rabbi Avraham Drandoff, Rabbi Avi Goldstein, Rabbi Henoch Millen, Rabbi Henoch Morris, Rabbi Effy Unterman, Rabbi Benyomin Weinschneider and Rabbi Howard Zack for your leadership in our community, your continued teachings of Torah, and for answering a multitude of questions.

Shimona Tzukernik for awakening my soul to *Chassidus*, helping me spread my dance to Jewish women everywhere, and for believing in me.

Rochelle L. Millen, PhD, for selfless hours of

editing and insightful, kind and gentle guidance.

Susan Berrin for her wisdom and expertise.

Beth Salzberg for a lifetime of friendship, support, and encouragement in my Torah growth.

Janice Cohen, who continues to hold a special place in my heart. Thank you for bringing yoga into my life when I needed it most.

Nancy Rapport for a listening ear, an eye for editing and humor when it is most needed.

To Angela Lamonte for holding the fort and doing so with a smile; and for your ongoing collegial advice and support.

Rabbi Yitzhok Adler and Leslie Adler for meeting me at the bottom of the ladder and helping me to climb it one rung at a time.

My brothers and sister: Rabbi Dovid Wachs, for refusing to give up on me and providing me with a lifetime of mentorship, love, and Beauchamp jokes. Steven Wachs for your love and support. Though we see the world so differently, we are able to respect and love one another. Ellen Wachs, whom I love just the way she is. Thank you for your belief in my abilities.

Lucinda Kirk, my writing partner, colleague and friend, for our serious, humorous, delightful writing sessions and therapy whenever I needed it, and to Bob Kirk for the shared writing sessions and thoughtful critique.

Jonathan Cassell for your help in editing this book and sharing your honest, unfiltered opinion.

My children Hana, Arielle, Leah, Daniel, Jon, and granddaughter Dahlia for filling my life with joy, purpose and laughter.

My husband Al, who has heard the same stories over and over again and yet remains my biggest fan. You are my rock, the love of my life, and my partner for life.

My parents for your unconditional love for me throughout my life, unending belief in my abilities and for your helpful warnings to watch out for the obelisks in all of my journeys.

My editor, Leslie Nolen, for gently but firmly lifting me out of my rut and onto the writing block and for keeping me going with expert guidance, accountability and humor.

Of course, to G-d, the Almighty who lifted me from the pit and caused my soul to dance (Psalm 30). You bring me to tears of joy and allow me to feel Your presence in all of my life.

I wish for each of you a life filled with joy and purpose, just as you have brought such light into mine.

About the Author

Author and teacher Shelly Dembe restores joyful purpose to everyday life, with inspiration, humor and practical lessons from her life as a young mom, free spirit, empty-nester and nurse who eventually traded the ICU for a yoga studio—only to find that the inner peace her soul sought in yoga was present in her Jewish faith all along.

She travels worldwide to Jewish communities as a facilitator of SefirotDance and speaker on physical and spiritual wellbeing and teaches classes and workshops in her home yoga studio.

Shelly is a registered nurse, holds the E-RYT 500 Yoga Alliance designation, and is a YogaDance Instructor certified by Kripalu, a certified LifeForce Yoga Practitioner for Anxiety and Depression, and a personal trainer certified by the American College of Sports Medicine.

She lives in Columbus, Ohio with her husband. Together they have four children and one grandchild.

Wrestling With Yoga

Journey of a Jewish Soul

Shelly Dembe

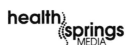

Table of Contents

Author's Note

I have chosen to represent our Creator's name throughout as G-d or Hashem to respect the holiness of G-d's name. Jews are not permitted to tear, destroy, or dispose of anything with G-d's name on it and this practice also guards against desecration of even the written Name through accidental destruction.

Generally, Hebrew and Sanskrit words are italicized and explained the first time they are used. Definitions are also found in the Glossary. Most Hebrew words are written in the Sephardic dialect because of its greater familiarity for most Jews. Exceptions to Sephardic usage are present in some quoted material and for certain words more commonly seen in the Ashkenazic style.

Introduction

Yoga *ashrams* across the globe are filled with Jews.

Sounds of Sanskrit emanate from the mouths of Jews who once recited Hebrew.

Thousands of Israelis flock to India every year in search of spiritual growth.

Yet, despite our Torah's cautions against idol worship, many of these same Jews are found bowing to deities displayed in yoga studios.

Many Jews experience spiritual feelings by simply attending yoga classes or by emptying the mind through meditation, forgetting the cautions against an empty mind.

One can find rabbis who condone the practice of yoga for physical health, and others who forbid it.

Are there clear guidelines for Jews who would like to practice yoga while still honoring their faith and its commandments?

This is the subject I will explore in this book.

An Unexpected Journey

I am often referred to as the "Jewish yoga lady." Go ahead and picture it: a tall, thin woman with a flowing colorful scarf on her head, stretchy cotton skirt over yoga pants, sitting in the lotus position and chanting *shalom.*

But being Jewish and doing yoga, as if they always went together, took years of struggle and searching to be able to dwell comfortably inside my eclectic being.

Like many Jews, I have wrestled with defining my Jewish identity. And even today, I choose not to limit my spiritual growth with labels associated with any particular set of Jewish practices.

I simply call myself what I most authentically am: an evolving Jew.

I am interested in sharing this struggle with you. Perhaps you are Jewish, Christian, Buddhist, or unaffiliated. You might be a yoga student who is curious about your faith, or an observant Jew wondering if yoga is permissible.

Yoga, meaning to unite or yoke, draws the body and soul together through a variety of practices. Even if one strictly practices yoga for physical benefit only, such as strength, flexibility or balance, the soul cannot be separated from the body in the physical world.

As students refine their practice, they may experience improved agility in the physical body, and confidence in the emotional realm. As obstructions are removed both physically and mentally, the soul can begin to speak its truth.

Garments of the Soul

In the language of the *Kabbalah*, the mystical teachings of the Torah, the soul is clothed by garments. These "garments of the soul" include thoughts, speech and actions.

What garments blanket the soul during yoga practice? Have we consciously chosen these garments to dress our inner selves?

These are questions I have been asking myself as a Jew, as a yoga teacher and student, and as someone whose soul yearns for an authentic, honest connection with my Creator.

In other words, I desire not only a healthy physical body, but a healthy soul as well, both in this world and in the world to come.

In no way am I suggesting that my beliefs should be your beliefs. I merely share my journey and continued struggle, both frustrating and enlightening, and encourage you to examine your own practices, beliefs and uncertainties.

Searching for Connection

I remember sitting in the hard pews of my childhood Reform Jewish temple, wanting so much to feel something; but instead I mostly thought about the chocolate eclairs I would indulge in at the *Oneg Shabbat*, the reception after the service. As my fingers flipped through the remaining pages of the prayer book, I tried to guess when the service would be over.

Movement consisted of standing and sitting only when the rabbi asked us to do so.

Even then, I had a desire to feel the prayers with my whole body and make some kind of spiritual connection. Hard as I tried to connect with something greater than the dessert selection, holy thoughts eluded me.

As I became an adult, I thought perhaps I lacked a connection because I had never celebrated my *bat mitzvah* at the age of 12 with any kind of party or ceremony. So as a young adult, I decided to reclaim this significant event.

Preparation for my group *bat mitzvah* included a rudimentary introduction to Hebrew, memorization of a few verses of the Torah which we would chant in front of the congregation, and participation in an Introduction to Judaism course.

We were also asked to compose a paper on any Jewish subject that piqued our curiosity. My choice? The search for spirituality in Reform Judaism. Scanning the Jewish libraries for juicy words of wisdom, I remained thirsty.

Inspired by their *bat mitzvah* ceremony, my classmates plunged into synagogue service, assuming various leadership roles.

But I still felt that something was missing. I had not found the closeness I craved.

Instead of experiencing connection with my colleagues and the congregation, I felt like a foreigner from a distant village.

While continuing to struggle with my place in Judaism, I wrestled in another arena, my marriage. As someone who loved fitness and movement, my hours in the gym distracted me temporarily but what I really wanted was spiritual comfort.

And that was when I turned to yoga.

As an athlete and personal trainer, I loved the physical challenge. Breathing practices helped calm me, mindfulness practice helped ground me, and meditation became my form of prayer.

Off to the *ashrams* I went, studying yoga philosophy, learning about my shortcomings and building confidence.

The more I took care of myself, the more the marriage crumbled. After a painful struggle to keep it going, we realized that our children were suffering as well. We ended our marriage, and our two children and I moved into a modest three-bedroom Colonial.

Down the street from our cozy new home stood a small friendly Orthodox *shul*—the Yiddish word for synagogue.

And just like that, the rabbi invited us to a Sabbath

dinner at his home. The Jewish Sabbath, also known as *Shabbat* or *Shabbos*, begins at sundown Friday and ends at sundown Saturday.

I began studying with him weekly. Before long, we were welcomed to the Sabbath tables of congregants we barely knew for savory food, song, and schmoozing.

Finding My Jewish Spark

So my life started to look and feel quite different: our home was feeling more peaceful, my job was joyful and fulfilling, and the beginnings of a Jewish spark began to light up our home.

When I think about this time period, I can picture my daughter Leah, then eight years old, covering her head with a lace cloth as she had seen me do on rare occasions. As she proudly stood next to me, she circled her hands around the Sabbath candles and attempted to say the appropriate blessing.

Joining her, I too began to say the blessing. Remembering how my mother would thank G-d after lighting candles, I began to speak out loud in thanks to G-d. My son Daniel listened with curious ears to my words of gratitude.

I wanted them to feel their faith inside their little bodies, to grow up believing in something greater than themselves, able to draw on the strength of G-d's presence when they needed to feel that spark that I had been searching so long for.

There were many other new sparks in our life:

walking to synagogue together on Saturday mornings, playing Monopoly in the afternoon, and becoming part of a new community whose members invited us to their homes for meals of matzoh ball soup and homemade challah.

There were also some hard realities, like major financial struggles as a single mom.

I remember pricing kitchen chairs and wondering how we were going to afford them when one day the kids and I were shopping at Walmart and there they were: four plastic chairs, $22 each; one lime green, one hot pink, one purple and one candy blue.

My children shrieked with delight and claimed the colored chair of their choice. The fourth chair remained empty for quite a while, occasionally filled by the boyfriend of the moment.

Finding My Other Half

As my Jewish practice grew, I started entertaining the idea of a future soulmate.

I had so much love to share, and I had grown to believe that I deserved a healthy, lifelong marriage.

Yet at 38, dating was a bit challenging.

After all, here I was: a "crunchy" and somewhat observant Jewish yogi.

Was there actually a match for me out there somewhere?

My rabbi suggested that I might begin praying for what I was seeking. I traded my early morning

Sanskrit chanting for Hebrew, and my new prayer book replaced my morning meditation.

Shortly thereafter, my catalog from the beautiful Kripalu yoga center arrived, and I noticed that Basherte, an organization that helps Jews meet their soulmates, was offering a weekend workshop at Kripalu.

Not having enough guts to sign up for Basherte's singles retreat, I signed up for a Kripalu yoga and dance program and went anyway. I had stayed there earlier during my YogaDance training, and to me it felt like home.

After one of my Kripalu classes that weekend, I met the Eisens, the organizers of Basherte. They discovered that I was Jewish, single, and a YogaDance teacher—and in no time, invited me to lead a dance at their Basherte retreat at Elat Chayyim, a Jewish retreat center in upstate New York.

At that retreat, as I pretended not to notice the plethora of single men all looking for Mrs. Right, the instructor placed me in front of my future husband for a mirroring exercise.

If that wasn't enough of a sign from G-d, the Basherte website matched us up as well, based on the attributes we had individually said mattered most: committed to Jewish values, emotionally open, physically active, joyful.

As I stared at the Basherte match on my computer, I wanted so much to believe that I was experiencing a miracle. After all, what was the likelihood of matching that closely with someone?

Our Jewish Brady Bunch

It didn't take us long to feel the hand of G-d in this relationship.

Our courtship was quick. We were married nine months after our first meeting at the Elat Chayyim retreat center. Amazingly, his two children and my two children became best of friends.

I'm sure you can picture it, our Jewish Brady Bunch: "It's the story, of a lovely lady..."

Our gratitude soared as we pinched ourselves to make sure it was all real. It was easy to take on more *mitzvot*, or commandments. It was our way of thanking G-d for our abundance.

Several years into this blissful marriage, we relocated to a city that was new for both of us.

Because of our growing observance, we moved into a neighborhood within walking distance of the Orthodox Jewish *shuls*.

The spacious living room in our new home became my first real yoga studio. No longer would I have to rent space where I could teach. No longer would I battle smells drifting from the church kitchen or intrusive sounds of the vacuum cleaner pushed by obedient custodians just doing their job.

With freshly laid bamboo floors and dreamy periwinkle blue walls, my studio welcomed students varied in faith, age and experience.

Showing up with—yes, you guessed it, a flowing and colorful scarf on my head—I began to share my yoga knowledge with students both in my studio and throughout the city.

The Jewish yogi in me was content. For a while.

1: Namaste

An Urge To Shout

The yoga studio is packed with students.

I can smell the sweat of the man next to me as he sits inches away, his skin slippery like a basted turkey on Thanksgiving.

The walls seem to vibrate to the rhythm of *ujayi* breaths, the ocean breaths of 40 or so people.

Our teacher asks us to bring our hands together in prayer position, in front of our chest. I hear a loud, echoing "Namaste!" from the mouths of all present, including me, followed by bows toward the floor and toward the teacher.

Ugh...at this moment I feel a knot in my stomach.

On my worn and familiar yoga mat in row six of

the packed classroom, I have the urge to shout out, "Who are you bowing to?"

Instead, I quietly and obediently roll up my mat, smile sweetly to the others around me, and take pleasure in the sensations of stretched muscles, calm breath, and breathable pores. Yes, I reassure myself, yoga is so good for me! And the bowing down...well, I'll just let that one go and leave it behind.

As a yoga student for over 20 years, I've always been taught that *namaste* could be translated as, "I honor the light within you." That is simply a lovely thought.

And in my Jewish mind, I reassure myself that we all hold the light of G-d within us. So why was it that every time I put my hands together in what's called "prayer position" and say *namaste* I feel an uncomfortable tugging at my Jewish soul?

At First, Delight

As the question became too loud to ignore, my investigations revealed deeper meaning behind the word *namaste*. *Namaste* is a Hindi salutation that combines two Sanskrit words, *nama* ("to bow") and *te* ("you"), into a greeting that translates roughly to "I bow to you."

Staring into the computer screen, my heart skipping, I'm experiencing an "aha" moment.

At first, my thought is one of delight, the way you feel when you find that second earring you've been missing.

But fear quickly replaced this feeling of discovery.

I am suddenly transported to the Reform temple of my childhood.

The rabbi in his booming voice brings to life the story of the golden calf. I remember my trepidation as I pictured the Jews of that time worshiping this animal, climaxing in the breaking of the tablets by Moshe, or Moses, in his fit of anger.

Though it was years before I really studied the prohibitions against idol worship, *avodah zorah*, and began to explore its manifestations, I always knew it was a sin.

The first commandment says, "I am the Lord thy G-d." It does not say "Gods." The second commandment says, "Thou shalt have no other gods before me."

We hear G-d's request that we worship only G-d, not the sun, moon, or a statue with three heads.

If we delve into our Torah, we see repeatedly how Jews were punished for praying to idols. In particular, when Moshe did not return from the mountain and the people became impatient, they built a golden calf, an idol made from their jewelry. We still suffer today as a people as a result of this incident.

And the *Shema*—familiar to nearly every Jew—proclaims "Hear, O Israel, the Lord is our G-d, the Lord is One. " Jews are instructed to cover their eyes and pronounce each word of this sacred prayer clearly and thoughtfully, indelibly engraving its meaning upon the soul.

As I brought these threads together, I could no longer rationalize bowing to the teacher, or indeed bowing at all while sitting. Jews are not to bow to anything or anyone other than G-d. Moreover, why was I, a Jew, using the language of a Hindu prayer?

Those who disagree with this line of thinking may feel that saying *namaste* is not problematic. One can have the intention to say it with the understanding that they are simply honoring the light in another.

But we all have different sensitivities.

For example, I have friends who can watch a violent or scary movie and feel unaffected by it. To them it is exciting and interesting. In my experience with such movies, I'm left feeling emotionally and physically distressed. The images do enter my body and pass into my soul, harming me, and thus I choose to avoid such films.

It is important to examine the effects our thoughts, words and actions have on our constitution.

We as Jews are commanded to study Torah and continue to evolve and grow closer to our Creator. Through this growth, we refine the garments of our soul.

In this moment of epiphany, I decided that I would not, could not, recite the word *namaste* even one more time.

My decision was made.

Now what?

Living With My Decision

As a yoga teacher for those of all faiths, including Jews of all affiliations, I knew an explanation would be necessary before simply leaving out this widely accepted salutation at the end of my yoga classes.

So the following day, after leading my students in postures, I explained that I had discovered another meaning for the salutation *namaste*. Explaining that *namaste* also means bowing down to another, which is incongruent with my faith, I asked my students to please refrain from bowing down to me as their teacher.

Today, I end all of my classes with *shalom* and I bring my hands onto my heart in a gesture of appreciation.

After all, peace for the hippie, Hindu, or Jew is a value few can wrestle with.

2: Chanting

Whoa, Nellie!

A swami, a Hindu master of yoga, attended our yoga training to enlighten us in yogic philosophy.

After sitting in meditation, we all drew each other close with chanting. All of the students seemed mesmerized by this communal vibration, with one exception.

I cautiously approached my teachers and hesitantly expressed a bit of reservation.

You see, by now I was used to standing out.

It was always something.

I was the one who could not eat the food everyone else enjoyed at yoga potlucks. Because I did not drive as part of my observance of Shabbat, Saturday workshops found me walking miles to the yoga studio, showing up looking like a drenched cat.

So I imagined my teachers saying impatiently to themselves: "What now?"

To my great relief, my honorable and respectable mentors assured me that chanting was optional. After class, I asked the swami to give me a copy of the chant, and I rushed home, eager to find out its meaning:

> "vande gurunam charanaravinde
>
> sandarsita svatmasukhava bodhe
>
> nihsreyase jangalikayamane
>
> samsara halahala mohasantyai
>
> abahu purusakaram
>
> sankhacakrasi dharinam
>
> sahasra sirasam svetam
>
> pranamami patanjalim
>
> om"

> *English translation:*

> "I bow to the lotus feet of the guru who awakens insight into the happiness of pure Being,
>
> who is the final refuge, the jungle physician,

who eliminates the delusion
caused by the poisonous herb of
samsara [conditioned existence]."

I prostrate before the sage
Patanjali

who has thousands of radiant,
white heads

[in his form as the divine serpent,
Ananta]

and who has, as far as his arms,
assumed the form of a man
holding a conch shell [divine
sound],

a wheel [discus of light,
representing infinite time]

and a sword [discrimination].

om"

Whoa, Nellie!

Stop this ride and let me get off!

Memories of my chanting in *ashrams*, yoga studios and even in my home practice came crashing into the shoreline of my mind.

A tsunami of fear washed over me.

What else had I proclaimed over the years, unknowingly?

Choosing, With Intention

Let's face it; yoga can be cultish at times.

We do what our yoga teacher tells us to do, often without question. Move this way, breathe that way, chant these words, and we do it just because we've heard how good yoga is for us, or we think our teacher knows best.

I'm certainly not suggesting that all teachers create cultish behaviors or that all students take on a subservient role. Thankfully, many teachers today believe that the yoga must serve the individual, and not vice-versa. This is what my *Viniyoga* training taught me and the majority of my fine, ethical mentors reinforced this principle.

Looking back on my days of Sanskrit chanting, I am surprised and, need I say, disappointed in myself.

Why did I chant words when I didn't know their meaning?

Are others curious about what they're singing as well?

A student deepens his or her yoga practice by becoming more aware of physical sensations, breath, and eventually its effect on the psyche and spirit.

I suggest that we, as evolving yoga students, scrutinize what enters and leaves our body.

Movements, words, and thoughts during our practice dress our soul. Observing the milieu we create during our practice is as much a part of our experience as an *asana*, breath or chant.

3: Sun Salutation

The sun salutation, familiar as the warm-up at the beginning of most yoga classes, involves twelve postures done in a flowing sequence, repeated three to five times.

As a yoga student and teacher for 20 years, my body knows the poses, the flow, the sequence, and the rhythm of this quite inviting practice. I don't have to think about what comes next. The repetition provides the same comfort as singing Don McLean's "American Pie"—I know it and do not even have to think. Alas, I enter a trance-like state, which is exactly what yoga's founders intended.

The goal of physical yoga is to remove enough bodily obstruction to sit comfortably, meditate, and ascend to *samadhi*, a state of intense focus and union with the Divine.

To determine if a sun salutation is at all problematic for Jews or Christians, let's look more closely at its origins.

The sun salutation, *surya namaskar*, is a common sequence of *asanas* whose origins lie in the worship of Surya, the Hindu sun god. *Namaskar*, like *namaste*, means "to bow to or adore."

When yoga arrived in the Western world in the late 19th century, its practice quickly became primarily physical, and the association between the sun salutation sequence and its origins in worship of a sun god quickly faded.

However, students grounded in monotheistic faiths may want to increase their consciousness regarding their intention when performing this series of movements.

Avoiding traditional sun salutations may at first feel like putting up an unnecessary fence. However, fences exist to protect us from danger.

One way to guard against any suggested worship of other gods might be to vary the warmup and move away from strict adherence to the prescribed set of poses that clearly define the sun salutation. By varying the movements, the student emphasizes a yoga practice that serves the individual, and not one in which the student serves the yoga.

Another safeguard might be to refrain from labeling one's warmup as a sun salutation and to avoid using the Sanskrit name *surya namaskar* which is even more suggestive of idol worship.

A beautiful alternative to saluting the sun in the morning can be found in our Jewish morning blessings.

Found in our *siddur*, or prayer book, is the beautiful *Elokai Neshama* prayer, recited among other blessings every morning:

> "My G-d, the soul You placed
> within me is pure. You created it,
> You fashioned it, You breathed it
> into me, You safeguard it within
> me, and eventually You will take
> it from me, and restore it to me
> in Time to come. As long as the
> soul is within me, I gratefully
> thank You, Hashem (a word for
> G-d meaning the Name), my G-d
> and G-d of my forefathers, Master
> of all works, Lord of all souls.
> Blessed are You, Hashem, Who
> restores souls to dead bodies."

Many prayers in Judaism may seem foreign to us, particularly if we didn't learn them in our childhood. Or possibly, when we've been reciting them for so long they've become mechanical.

Elokai Neshama plants the seeds of renewal and restoration in our hearts and minds. Gratitude of our alive soul then permeates our physical body as we begin our physical yoga practice. Our focal point becomes not the sun, but our living and eternal G-d.

4: Modeh Ani

Students come to my home yoga studio to relax, re-energize, improve their flexibility, get stronger, lose weight, gain weight, learn how to breathe, be present, be happier, get a break from responsibility, get inspired, reduce anxiety...and so on.

The very first tool I teach them is how to center, better known as mindfulness. Yoga, which actually means to "yoke together," is the blending of body and mind. In other words, my mind is where my body is.

So we sit or lie down and notice where we are. We observe what is happening with our bodies, our minds, and our breathing.

I offer new students these guidelines to help them establish the centering process as a natural part of their practice:

How To Center Yourself

1. Schedule five minutes daily for centering. Let others know not to disturb you. Turn off your cell phone. Give yourself permission to step away from activity.

2. Sit comfortably with spine lengthened, on floor with pillow or blanket under you or in a straight-back chair.

3. Close your eyes.

4. Begin to relax the outer body. Quiet the movement of the eyes. Relax your jaw and tongue. Let the shoulders descend away from the ears. Release the arms and legs. Allow the body to unravel and soften.

5. Observe your breath. Become aware of where the breath moves in your body. Is it shallow or deep? Begin to deepen your breath. Inhale completely and slowly, exhale all of the air out.

6. Let go of the breath and focus on your mind. Let go of all thoughts of the past or future. Bring your mind to the present moment.

7. Allow gratitude to enter your heart as you appreciate this new moment in your life. Take notice of the miraculous nature of your body, the heart beating, the breath moving, the organs functioning.

8. Ask for an intention: what do I want to receive? What do I want to let go of? How am I feeling? Listen for the answer.

9. Use this centering at least once a day or anytime you need to refocus, recharge, or relax. Enjoy!

Jews are given the gift of centering every morning, and a structure to guide them. It is called *Modeh Ani*, and comes in the form of a prayer that is said upon awakening, even before we creep out of our cozy covers and step onto the bedroom floor.

> "Modeh anee lifanecha melech
> chai vikayam, she-he-chezarta
> bee nishmatee b'chemla, raba
> emunatecha.
>
> I offer thanks to You, living
> and eternal king, for You have
> restored my soul within me; Your
> faithfulness is great."

There it is: the acknowledgment of the soul alive in the body. A gift of another day has just been given to me. My Creator is alive and with me today!

Practicing With Grace

The yoga mat has not yet been rolled out, and already I am in my practice, loyal to my Jewish soul.

This practice extends gracefully into the creation of an intention for one's day. What is my purpose today? What tasks or activities will support my values?

Do I have so much on my plate that it will be impossible to focus on what really matters?

I may give myself permission to delegate, back off, or redirect my energy to honor what I really value.

Before I knew about *Modeh Ani*, my centering did not occur until I sat down on my yoga mat, and then only on days that I had a yoga practice.

Once the alarm clock went off, it was a race to accomplish as much as possible in the first minutes of the morning, before my children woke up. Or, if the kiddies woke me before my alarm clock did, my focus would immediately shift to their needs.

Modeh Ani allows us to thank G-d for our life and our living breathing soul, which is renewed every waking day...to start our days with a moment in a quiet, calm place before we enter the hubbub that is our day.

5: Meditation

Finding My Fix

Long before I discovered the daily Jewish practice of formal prayer, I probed into the pockets of gurus, looking for goodies.

As a chocoholic rampages through cupboards to uncover a morsel of the sweet dark stuff, I too wanted my fix.

You know the feeling: full but not satisfied. You eat everything but dessert, and then, finally throwing your hands up, you give in and just have what you tried so hard to resist. Then, at last, you can move on.

Well, I wanted that feeling of satiety in my life.

I remember attending a meditation class at a very large yoga conference. Before this class, I always told myself that meditation was out of the question. I just could not do it. I would never be one of those people who could just sit and empty my mind.

But here I was, in a conference room of 100 students ready to prove myself wrong. Our teacher suggested that for the first five minutes, we allow any thoughts to enter our mind and then kindly ask each thought to leave, without engaging in it. And so, I dismissed each idea that tickled my brain, making room for the next distraction, which of course was there, waiting in line for an appointment.

For the next five minutes of the meditation, our leader asked us to use a mantra—a word or phrase to repeat to ourselves. I spent the entire time trying to think of an appropriate repetition. The last five minutes were spent emptying the mind, and returning to the mantra if we found we were getting distracted by outside thoughts.

After that class, I went home and began a strict meditation practice. I ordered a *zafu*, a firm pillow for sitting on while meditating. I found pleasure in the empty spaces between the mantra. My busy thoughts became a pat of butter melting into a piece of toast.

I had arrived—or so I thought.

Despite my intention to allow the yoga to serve me, I obediently filled the prescription and took the daily yoga medicine ordered by the teacher of the moment. I started to notice a theme when attending yoga conferences. Each teacher thought his or her prescribed method was the best way to practice, and unless we followed each individual instructor's guidelines we would not grow in yoga.

How could each teacher be right? My frustration grew as I tried to hear my own voice through the barrage of yogic advice.

A Restless Soul Searches

My worlds of yoga and Judaism once again collided while attending a Jewish retreat in the mystical mountains of Tannersville, New York.

Allow me to set the scene for you.

My friend of many years had tried her best to convince me to attend *Kabbalah* authority Shimona Tzukernik's summer Jewish retreat in Tannersville. "It will really speak to you, Shelly," Beth insisted.

Perhaps I wasn't listening. Perhaps I wasn't ready for such change in my thinking. Whatever the reason, it took many years of persuasion and an invitation to teach yoga to finally get me to show up.

 You could say I've been climbing the Jewish ladder, one *mitzvah* at a time for the past ten years, adding a hop to my step this past year.

Occasional classes on Jewish thought, laws and practice with various teachers had given me more knowledge and understanding, but I was restless for more—more passion, more depth, and more connection.

I wanted to feel tingling under my skin.

Choosing to travel by car, the long drive from my home in Columbus, Ohio to Tannersville provided comfort and familiarity for my questioning soul.

However, after eleven hours of sitting in a confined space, I was ready to get out and explore. Into Shimona's house I strolled, to find a pair of warm, smiling eyes and a face surrounded by light.

"I know this face!" my soul exclaimed. It is the face of a fellow Jew, one with a shared connection to the Divine spark. And then there was my old, dear friend by my side, *kvelling* with joy as her circle of friends expanded yet again.

After settling into my cottage, my first job was to lead participants in a yoga session. So far so good; this was comfortable territory.

With words inviting all to be present, I too gave myself permission to breathe into this new moment. Daily yoga sessions would ground me in the familiar, and I could share my gifts of abundant health and movement with those needing comfort in their bodies.

Moving from meditation to a morning meal, I was then nourished by my new friend Miriam's conscious cooking. A bowl of creamy fresh oatmeal topped with earthy crunchy granola and juicy blueberries satisfied my taste buds and my healthy eating shtick. With a relaxed body and full belly, I curiously approached the makeshift classroom situated on the wraparound wooden porch.

Like a fleece jacket on a cool, crisp morning, the words of *Chassidus* that I heard that day warmed my flesh. These Hasidic teachings began revealing the mystical aspects of the Torah to my questing mind.

"'Sanctity of life' is a household term. But do we really know what that means? And do we as a society subscribe to the concept in actuality?" Shimona prodded.

"The value of life is connected to the contribution one makes to society," came one reply.

Before I could verbally reject this statement, Shimona intervened, assuring us that this interpretation is rejected by Jewish values. Whew!

She then captured my attention with the thought that "physical life is the connection of the Godly soul and the body. Murder is the premature separation of body and soul."

Poetic, inspiring lessons continued to flow from Shimona, like the metaphoric fountain of water she spoke of which flowed from her heart and nourished her twins at birth. She was now a wellspring for her students who would drink in her words in the days to come.

Afternoons found us close to the earth, inhaling the green growth of the forest as we ascended mountaintops. The children amongst our group skipped over roots and rocks, encouraging others with older bodies to enjoy the journey.

I found a new friend among these children: a three-year-old boy with blond curly locks and sparkly hazel eyes. His little hand grasped mine as we skipped from rock to rock.

You know three-year-olds. They've not yet learned how to filter their words, thus allowing delightfully unscreened thoughts to escape. Before taking a sip from his water bottle he called out proudly the blessing over the water.

> "Blessed are You, Lord our G-d,
> King of the universe, by Whose
> word all things came to be."

Curious to know if he knew why he was saying this blessing, I just asked him.

His reply? "Because G-d is in the water."

And I wondered. Who was helping who up this mountain?

Arriving at a vista, our eyes rested upon cities too far away to feel their pulse. Bird songs drew our attention to the mountaintops, quieting the chatter in our minds. We moved into our hearts and felt the camaraderie amongst us take root. Our Jewish souls feasted on our connection to each other and to G-d's artistry.

On our last day, Shimona defined happiness as "a state of being that arises from the awareness of the oneness of G-d."

Here it was: a definition so familiar to me. After all, the *Shema*, a proclamation of the Oneness of G-d, was the one prayer I knew from childhood.

Sitting in the pews of my Reform temple, I had recited this watchword of our faith every week.

Happiness had always been there for the taking and here it was at the retreat, the fountain quenching my thirst.

On the long ride home, I was grateful for the cocoon of the car which protected me from distraction. From Tannersville to Columbus, I soaked in the feeling of oneness with G-d.

Chassidus, in Shimona's words, teaches the heart to think and the mind to feel. I could feel the blood flowing through my body. My heart skipped with joy. And I could feel the tingling under my skin.

I was falling in love.

Putting Meditation In Its Place

Well, I floated for quite awhile after that retreat.

Until one morning, while sitting on my *zafu*, a feeling of unease crept into my meditation.

What had a senior teacher at the retreat said about meditation? She had cautioned me against emptying my mind.

Yes, that was it. With a stern voice and serious gaze, she let me know in no uncertain terms that Jews are cautioned against meditating to emptiness.

I felt like a small child scolded by the principal for misbehaving.

And in the immature part of my psyche that does not like to be reprimanded, I immediately discarded this idea. Who does she think she is? What does she know about yoga? She must be a religious fanatic.

And so I dismissed her warnings against meditation.

But why was I still squirming uncomfortably on

my *zafu*?

As we grow in our yoga practice, our senses become heightened. We may notice sensations that eluded us in the past. Students often begin yoga in order to manifest a change in their outer physical body. With time, they notice more subtle reactions under the skin, in the mind, and even in the spiritual realm.

Perhaps it was time to delve into the practice of meditation from a Jewish perspective. Perhaps there was truth to the teacher's warnings.

I began my research by turning to the wisdom of our Jewish teachers.

Rabbi Aryeh Kaplan's book *Jewish Meditation* illustrates the history, structure and purpose of meditation in Judaism. This book is an excellent guide for Jews who wish to understand and practice meditation safely.

Many Jews have left the traditional structure of Jewish practice, seeking alternative ways to satiate spiritual hunger, particularly through a more Eastern approach to meditation.

As Rabbi Kaplan of blessed memory points out, meditative practices among differing faiths may look quite similar. However, the desired outcomes can be quite varied.

Although Jewish prophets clearly entered mystical, meditative states through prayer and prophecy, Jewish leaders made a conscious decision to move away from mystical forms of meditation during the 1800s out of a concern that it could lead to idolatrous practices.

The *Amidah*, also known as the *Shemonah Esrei*, was composed in the fifth century. The Ba'al Shem Tov, founder of Hasidic Judaism in the early 1700's, encouraged all Jews to use the recitation of the *Amidah* as a safe form of meditation. Rabbi Kaplan also encourages modern Jews to use the *Amidah* as a mantra.

However, many Jews still find it difficult to keep one's mind on the words of the prayer. Rabbi Nachman, the great-grandson of the Ba'al Shem Tov, thus encouraged Jews to prepare for meditation by reciting other psalms and prayers prior to reciting the *Amidah*. This narrowing of one's thoughts would hopefully quiet the mind in preparation for standing before G-d.

By repeating a word, phrase or visualization, the practitioner is able to narrow the mind's focus, direct the mind toward the mantra, and control the mind's susceptibility to distractions.

Once we can begin to regulate our minds, we can increase our concentration.

If we continue along this path of increased awareness, we can then experience deeper meaning in our lives by understanding with greater clarity what Rabbi Kaplan terms "truths." For example, we may contemplate our purpose on this earth, the existence of G-d, or how to love another being when we don't like them. Ultimately, we may come to feel G-d's presence and Oneness.

In Jewish meditation, we use practices that lead us toward this goal of being in the presence of G-d. With the knowledge that G-d exists and we are all children of G-d, we can then strive to live a life honoring our Creator.

For example, if I am writing this book in order to satisfy my ego, I will be elated to find out that my book earned me a certain amount of money with which to buy new things.

I may enjoy the publicity I receive and feel pregnant with pride at my accomplishments. While there is nothing wrong with enjoying wealth or success, perhaps there is a deeper satisfaction to be found as well.

Through long hours of research, contemplation, and yes, meditation on the material I'm writing about, I'm discovering truths about myself and my faith.

I'm hopefully connecting with other Jews worldwide who might be struggling with similar thoughts. My own prayer practice may heighten as I learn techniques to focus on deeper meanings in our liturgy.

With increased *parnasah* (livelihood), I can be more generous with *tzedakah* (charity), and help support my children while they are studying Torah.

Back in my days on the *zafu*, I strove to free my mind of distractions in order to feel a sense of inner bliss. As a runner, my hours of movement allowed me to clear my mind and experience a more relaxed state. As a Jew, these qualities are valuable as well.

But what is the next step? What do we do with the gifts of a relaxed mind and body? Where does the ego stop calling the shots, allowing G-d to step in?

I've talked about the danger of serving others in the practice of yoga. We as students must internalize our practice and listen to our own needs.

Through Jewish meditation we can take our practice to the next step by meditating on what G-d wants from us.

When I began exploring *halacha*, Jewish scriptural laws that include keeping kosher, observing the Sabbath, and following the laws of family purity and the *mikvah*, I remember picking and choosing the laws that made sense to me, and discarding those that I could not digest.

My focus was on what my ego felt was important.

Rarely did I ask myself, "What does G-d want?"

When we ask ourselves if something makes sense to us, we are dwelling in the intellectual. Meditation is about leaving this rational state and entering a more subconscious arena. Here we can feel what we cannot articulate.

Living Meditations: Shabbat

Our Torah states that the Jews at Mt. Sinai heard the lightning and saw the thunder, proclaiming "Naaseh v' nishmah...We will do and we will learn." The order of these words tells us that first we act in accordance with the word of G-d, and only then do we understand the meaning and purpose of those actions.

The *mitzvot*, or commandments, are gifts from G-d. Observing and participating in such beautiful *mitzvot* allows us to draw closer to G-d.

I believe that my lifelong search for meaning in my Judaism took me to *ashrams* and yoga studios because I wanted to feel more connected to my Creator.

When I took on Jewish commandments like Shabbat, *kashrut* (keeping kosher), and *taharat hamishpacha* (the laws of family purity), I started to find the relationship that before had always eluded me.

Before observing the Sabbath, Saturday was just another day to run around and *do*...errands, laundry, work, exercise, the usual daily activities.

As the saying goes, "I was a human doing, not a human being." I could not imagine turning off for a day.

I loved my Saturday morning workout, answering email, and checking out the sales at a variety of stores. Even if I decided to relax, I wanted it to be my choice.

It was not until I actually experienced many *Shabbats*, or Sabbaths, that I felt the beauty of being instead of doing.

The practice of un-doing led me to the meditative experience of the Sabbath, where my day was filled with prayer, reading Jewish texts, and guiltless naps in my overstuffed chair.

Friday night and Saturday Sabbath meals created space to linger with friends. Ritual blessings were made over food, wine and light. Song and talks of Torah elevated our table. The *shechina*, or female energy, of the Divine presence was palpable. The commitment to a weekly observance of Sabbath allowed the Divine to enter our external and internal environment.

Living Meditations: Keeping Kosher

Eventually, our Sabbath rituals led me to a new consideration of *kashrut*, the act of keeping kosher.

Jews who observe *kashrut* must meditate on what they're putting into their bodies before they buy and eat food.

This practice resonated with me. As a registered nurse and personal trainer, I've always carried a passion for healthy food. In fact, my dedication to pure, wholesome food is well known among family and community members. Friends frequently confess their eating sins to me, hoping that their confession to eating a pan of brownies will erase the calories ingested.

Congregants at synagogue events peek at my plate, wondering if I'll indulge in the conventional meat stew, *cholent*.

Fortunately, my daughter laughs whenever she shares her memory of my outburst at the Good Humor truck. It was a terribly hot day in West Hartford, Connecticut, the kind of hot that makes a barefoot child hop across the scorching pavement as if it were coals.

What could be more exciting to an overheated child than the musical jingle of the ice cream truck, beckoning parents to emerge from their homes, wallets in hand?

The part of me that had fond memories of my own childhood dates with vanilla-orange pushups wanted to bolt out of my house and watch my children deliberate over the many treats pictured on the side of the large white van.

My daughter chose a crunchy coated bar with a chocolate-filled center. My son, not usually one for sweets, opted for a monster green popsicle. While helping him remove the wrapper, my rational brain zeroed in on the ingredients as I watched his mouth turn dreadful colors.

As much as I tried to restrain myself so that they could just enjoy this infrequent pleasure, I found myself shouting, "Chemicals on a stick...that's what this is!"

I even went so far as to submit an article to the local paper, asking the world why ice cream trucks couldn't offer real ice cream. Was it so hard to replace propylene glycol and red #40 with eggs, milk, sugar and real fruit flavors?

I will no longer belabor the point; let's just say I had and continue to have strong feelings about what I put into my physical body.

And yet, despite this, I was questioning the value

and necessity of keeping kosher. I was mindful about what the kiddies ate, and what went into my mouth, yet I still felt resistance.

As a devoted yogi, I appreciated the food prepared for me. I acknowledged the many people who worked hard to ensure I had fresh food, including the farmers, the store owners, and whoever cooked my meal. I even took a minute to focus on my plate and its abundance before I put fork to mouth.

And yet, the commandment of eating strictly kosher food eluded me. As one who prided herself on being flexible off the yoga mat as well as on it, I valued eating at friends' homes and enjoying the food from other cultures while traveling to foreign cities.

Keeping kosher would change our vacation experiences, limit our social dining experiences, and decrease our repertoire of culinary delights.

Bluntly, I could not imagine giving up succulent butter-drenched lobster!

The laws of *kashrut* are known as *chukkim*—rules that do not have a rationale. We are to obey them simply to follow G-d's commandment. However, humans seek meaning in all they do, and so I found a deeper purpose in adhering to the kosher laws.

As the common saying goes, "We are what we eat." It pleased me greatly to learn that birds of prey and animals who kill other animals for food are unkosher. Shellfish and water creatures who eat the scum off the ocean floor are also unfit for Jewish consumption.

Historically, Jews were given permission to eat

meat as a concession to their weaknesses. Many Jews today turn away from meat and choose vegetarianism as a vehicle for greater spiritual elevation.

Others have refined their definition of *kashrut* to include foods that are certified as ethically-produced and environmentally conscious by the Magen Tzedek Commission. Producers of *magen tzedek* foods follow ethical standards for treatment of workers and animals, comply with worker safety standards, and use environmentally-conscious production methods.

With this deeper purpose, what first felt like a deprivation became another type of meditation, a greater connection to my Creator. Narrowing my focus to adhere to laws greater than myself created a new consciousness around eating, an activity most of us partake in at least three times a day.

Putting my ego aside once again, I enjoyed the discipline of this commandment. Eating in this way nourished not just my physical body, but my soul as well.

Living Meditations: Family Purity

The *mitzvah* of *mikvah, taharat hamishpacha*, the laws of family purity that address the relationship between husband and wife, is another example of a living meditation that creates space and connection, two goals of meditation.

Sex in our society has permeated our environment, degrading an act meant to create intimacy, life, and connection with our Creator. Billboards feature body parts not normally uncovered. Sitcoms geared for families with young children routinely include sexual scenarios, and even candy commercials are laced with sexual innuendos.

The result of this sexual freedom is a numbing of our senses; a movement away from the sacred. We as Jews have been blessed by G-d to protect our souls and preserve our relationships with our spouses. Our Torah provides a safeguard against the idolatry that abounds in worshipping bodies that do not belong to us.

Mikvah, just one element of this intricate *mitzvah*, both protects a relationship and provides space for the sacred in a marriage. For example, during a woman's menses, husband and wife refrain from physical contact with each other. After her menses cease, husband and wife avoid physical contact for an additional seven days, creating a separation for approximately two weeks.

During this time, couples are encouraged to strengthen their communication with each other in ways outside of the physical.

Once this period of time ends, the woman immerses herself in a *mikvah*, a holy body of water, and her spiritual status changes from spiritually impure to spiritually pure.

She and her husband are now able to reunite. Couples often feel a sense of renewal and appreciation for each other.

This *mitzvah* is not without its challenges, yet for

many couples it creates physical and emotional space for each spouse, heightening the connection with each other and elevating the relationship.

Living Meditations: In Service To Others

Plenty of other rituals and commandments in Judaism provide opportunities for living meditation as well.

Tikkun olam, translated as "repairing the world," is a value integral to Judaism and practiced by the vast majority of Jews today. Examples include volunteer work, giving charity, and engaging in social action.

The parallel in the yoga world is *karma* yoga or *seva*, service to others, an element frequently found at yoga retreats and one I admire.

After spending time focusing on oneself for a few days at a retreat, the organizers will often schedule a volunteer task for participants.

I hold today a beautiful memory of such an experience. Our local yoga studio offered a summer getaway in the quiet farmlands of southern Ohio. We were treated to early morning yoga in an earthy yurt, silent walks in a labyrinth made of tall grass, and homemade oatmeal raisin cookies that graced cups of steaming hot tea.

After two days of basking in these peaceful surroundings, we were given an opportunity to give back to those who prepared such a lovely space for us.

After choosing from a list of tasks, we were instructed to work together for two hours in silence. While I and several other students washed windows, we enjoyed the silent camaraderie. It was truly a living meditation of thanks.

One need not practice yoga or attend a yoga retreat in order to experience a living meditation.

When we create the right intention, beginning in our minds, our soul can meditate.

Melanie, a petite Filipino woman with bright eyes and a skip in her step, helps put the sparkle in my home. As she dusts and vacuums, she hums a tune, stopping every so often to share an insight with me. As a devout Christian, she spends her evenings in prayer and song, and her days infusing love into her work. Despite a life of hardship, she feels gratitude for where she is today. Her work has become a living meditation.

Grateful for where I am today as well, I cannot say I am sorry for the time spent on my *zafu* in the rooms of the *ashrams*. My training in mindfulness helps me daily to live with awareness of what is in front of me, whether it's a beautiful flower, a friend in need of being heard, or a new challenge to face.

When praying, I appreciate the importance of emptying my mind of extraneous thoughts in order to connect to my Creator.

And through this exploration of meditation in Judaism, I realize the vastness of this subject, barely touched by my mind.

6: Om

Aaaaaa...Ooooo....Mmmmm

When written, "aaaaaa...oooooo....mmmmm"
resembles the sounds made by a crowd at a
spectacular Fourth of July fireworks display.

But put it all together and you get *om*, a Sanskrit
vibration emanating from yoga studios around the
world.

Yoga teachers are taught that *om* is the universal
vibrational sound of the earth. *Om*-ing is a way to
bring a group together at the beginning of a class,
and to end a class as well. It seemed to me at some
of my trainings that we *om*'d before and after every
sentence.

For a while, I *om*'d along with the group,

wondering if I was the only one feeling uncomfortable. Was I being ridiculous? Everyone else claimed to feel unified. Instead, I felt isolated.

Then one day it dawned on me that *om* was the ending sound of *shalom*. So I decided in the privacy of my mind to chant *shalom* when everyone else said *om*. No one needed to know.

And my discomfort calmed for awhile.

But as usual, my questing mind led to further explorations.

Wikipedia defines *om* as a mystical Sanskrit sound which is considered sacred by Hindus, Sikhs, Buddhists and Jains.

It is placed at the beginning of most Hindu texts as an incantation to be intoned at the beginning and end of a reading of the sacred Hindu texts, the Vedas, and before any prayer. *Om* represents an invitation to the god being worshipped to partake in the sacrifice.

I'll admit that chanting can be a unifying experience. After all, when we reflect on the garments of the Jewish soul, we learn how powerful speech is. The vibration created by a communal sound like *om* enters the body and stimulates the senses.

However, neither Judaism nor Christianity appear among the religions mentioned in the discussion of *om*. We of monotheistic faith are not instructed to invoke gods.

Fortunately, we have in our own practice safe ways to experience unifying vibrations. In fact, Judaism is filled with beautiful moving prayers and songs to uplift and connect us.

The *niggun* is a Jewish song composed of sounds rather than words or formal lyrics. Traditionally they are sung in groups and repeated over and over. In Hasidic circles, this form of meditative prayer set to wordless repetitive melody is designed to evoke a state of *devekut*, feelings of intense joy and of a clinging to G-d during prayer.

Devekut is also used to describe a state of deep meditation accessed through Torah learning, engagement in *mitzvot*, and as discussed here, through repetitive chanting.

Regular attendance at Jewish houses of worship like *shuls*, synagogues, and temples can provide a searching soul a place to connect with community. Singing at a Sabbath meal draws those at the table closer.

Saturday afternoons often find my husband and me back at *shul* for a light afternoon meal followed by singing. The leader, in a strong, melodic voice, leads us in the prayerful song *Mizmor L'David*, translated as:

> "A Psalm of David.
>
> The Lord is my shepherd, I shall not want. He lays me down in green pastures, He leads me beside still waters.
>
> He restores my soul. He leads me on the path of justice for His Name's sake. Though I walk

through the valley of the shadow
of death, I will fear no evil, for
You are with me.

Your rod and Your staff, they
comfort me.

You prepare a table before me in
view of my enemies. You anoint
my head with oil, my cup runs
over.

May only goodness and kindness
follow me all the days of my life.

May I live in the House of the
Lord forever."

The lyrics are sung in Hebrew, and even though I
do not know the exact translation, I am moved by the
melody. I also feel an unspoken connection to those
around me, though I may not know them all.

On Saturdays when we do not make it back to *shul*,
my husband and I sing together around our dining
room table. Like a lover's embrace, we hold on to our
Sabbath during the last remaining hour and celebrate
with song...an intimate moment with my husband
and with my Creator.

It's not clear to me whether yogic practices such as
chanting and *om*-ing are dangerous. How does a Jew
really know what is problematic?

Deepening Our Faith

Using *om* as an example, I am suggesting that we as Jews search for vehicles for connection and preparation in our yoga practice by looking within the framework of Jewish practice.

In this way, we veer away from practices that were designed for those of other belief systems, as we grow in Jewish knowledge.

On a broader scale, we as Jews are to be a light to the nations. Clear expression of Jewish values through our own Jewish practices shows others that we are collectively strong at a time when our cultural and spiritual identity may be diminishing.

Alan Dershowitz in *The Vanishing American Jew* states that "American Jewish life is in danger of disappearing, just as most American Jews have achieved everything we ever wanted: acceptance, influence, affluence, equality."

Ironically and sadly, it was anti-Semitism that historically provided the fuel for many Jews to fight back, clinging to their faith with intense fervor. History holds stories of women sneaking in the dark to hidden *mikvahs* and of bearded men with holy books whispering words of Talmud in unknown corners.

The need to stand together, to assert our right to openly practice our religion, dwindles when we no longer have guns held to our heads. Jews today do not generally have to resist blatant persecution as we have in the past. Yet ironically, with all the freedom we have to embrace our Jewish practice, many choose to assimilate into cultures and faiths that feel less confining.

The freedom that abounds in the Jewish world today gives us greater permission to ask why.

Why should I continue a ritual that my ancestors practiced? *Chukkim*, as mentioned earlier, are commandments for which there is no logical reason, such as *kashrut*. It is easy to forgo this *mitzvah* which lacks a sensible rationale, and enjoy the status of acceptance, influence, affluence, and equality as quoted above, not to mention pleasure in eating whatever we darn well please, or dining in the most talked-about restaurant in town.

As I go off on a philosophical tangent, hang in there with me. I will wrap it up neatly in a few paragraphs.

Om-ing for yogis is as mainstream as the sampling of gastronomic delights for foodies. Why not *om* and join the ranks of most in doing so to share in a universal vibration?

Through this communal chant, we are bringing disparate parts into one: many students together into one voice. And each participant experiences the oneness singly as well, narrowing the focus of each toward an inner sense of peace.

According to Janani Cleary, Hindu scholar and author of "OM: Its Purpose and Meaning," the purpose of *om*-ing is "to attach oneself to the god that pervades the universe." *Om* unites the individual with the Divine.

In Judaism, however, our Torah provides us with a direct path back to the beginning of time. Intermediaries are not used to reach G-d. Talmudic scholar Rabbi Eliyahu Eliezer Dessler's *Strive for Truth* explains that *chukkim*, laws without clear rational reasons, provide us the opportunity to draw very close to G-d.

Mishpatim, laws which can be understood rationally, allow Jews to adhere to laws which are based on easily comprehended intellectual principles. For example, the commandment, "Thou shall not steal" is easy and logical to understand.

On the other hand, laws of *kashrut*, keeping kosher, lack this easy understanding. A Jew may observe these laws simply out of fear or awe of G-d.

I mentioned earlier in this chapter the concept of *devekut*, a state of attachment to G-d which can be accessed through the repetitive singing of *niggunim*, or wordless melodies. *Devekut*, which is literally translated as "a clinging," represents a state in which we feel attached to our Creator as well as to all beings.

This lofty level necessitates a complete surrender to the Oneness and completeness of G-d. Reasoning is discarded and the Jew is embraced by nothing but G-d.

May we as Jews reach out to receive this embrace not by chanting *om*, but by following the channels set out for us by our own Creator.

7: Sacred Music

Nirvana In The Sunrise Studio

The Kripalu Center for Yoga houses the sunrise studio where the morning sunlight streams into the eastern windows.

I am lying on a mat directly in line with one of these rays, feeling the warmth on my face as I lie in *savasana*, the lying-down pose at the end of class.

Also pouring into the room is an incredibly beautiful sound, that of Deval Premal singing "Om Namo Bhagavate Vasudevaya," a Hindu mantra.

I find the melody intoxicating, and I want to drink it in along with the warm rays of the sun. It is one of the most rapturous sounds I have ever heard. I must download this music and use it in my teaching, I promise myself.

During the course of my stay at Kripalu, I continue to be drawn to the rhythmic music. I feel like a baby who is being swaddled and rocked by her mother.

Music has always affected me in a deep way. It is almost impossible for me to sit still when music is in the air, whether it's James Brown or Beethoven.

It was a natural progression for me to become a certified YogaDance instructor, and in doing so, I attended the Kripalu Center for an extended period of time.

Through the expertise of fine yoga teachers like Megha and Nateshvar, we learned to express the *chakras*, or wheels of energy in the body, through dance. Each *chakra* held an emotion that we aimed to evoke through a specific type of music.

The first *chakra*, root *chakra*, involved drumming, earthy music to create the intention of grounding oneself.

In the second *chakra*, we used sensual music to encourage flowing, watery movements.

The remaining five *chakras* were expressed through movements elicited by a variety of music. The raspy voice of John Mellencamp belting out "When the walls come tumblin' down" created a fervor of foot-stomping among students in the vast chapel room.

I purchased Deva Primal's blissful CD in the incense-filled bookshop and eagerly read the liner notes, which explained that "Om Namo Bhagavate

Vasudevaya" translated to "prostration to Krishna" or "surrender to Krishna." Those of Hindu faith believe that Krishna himself asked his devotees to completely surrender to him by reciting this mantra daily.

Other songs paid homage to Lord Vishnu and asked listeners to bow down to deities. Also included in the CD were songs speaking of universal peace and love.

I decided to leave behind the intoxicating music of Deva Primal, turning to safer genres of music for my fix.

Today I choose from a variety of instrumental music as a background for my yoga classes. To facilitate the dances I lead, I draw from the wealth of soul-stirring Jewish music available today, with the addition of instrumental drumming sounds. For example, a favorite song requested by Jews and non-Jews alike is "*Oseh Shalom*," meaning "he who makes peace." An exquisite rendition is sung by the artist Yofiyah in the form of a chant.

Music is a powerful tool, evoking emotion, movement, and reflection. Judaism asks us to filter what we ingest, be it food, conversation or song.

8: Opening the Vessel

October 17, 1989

She must have been happy in there. It was warm, cozy, quiet.

But I was ready to meet her.

After 27 grueling hours of labor, Pitocin, and finally the forceps, Dr. Rutman and three nurses finally released Leah from my body's grip.

There she was, calm, pink, and mine.

"I know you!" I thought to myself.

Her face seemed so familiar to me, as if we had been friends for years.

She looked at me, I looked at her, and instinctively, I put her to my breast. She knew what to do. Her little mouth started sucking and once again she was attached to me.

All of a sudden I began to feel labor pains again. Wait a minute, I thought. Labor is supposed to be over! Then the doctor explained to me that when a baby nurses, the mother's uterus contracts. As a nurse, I appreciated the wonder of the human body. Working on cadavers in anatomy class taught me the complexity of organs, muscles and bones, all perfectly placed. Following a drop of blood through the circulatory system in physiology studies helped me visualize the necessity of open vessels.

And now, I was enlightened by the reciprocal relationship of mother and child.

With G-d's plan, I help give life to my baby and in turn, my infant helps to restore life to my tired body.

My awareness of G-d soared in that miraculous moment.

The Master of the Universe created me. He orchestrated the workings of my physical body like a symphony playing harmonious music. The instruments and the musicians compose the orchestra, but it is the conductor who brings out the balanced sounds of the concerto.

My days as a nurse in the busy cardiac ICU ended after Leah was born. I wanted more flexibility in my schedule, and so I moved on to cardiac rehabilitation and eventually into personal training and then to yoga. Much of my working day focused on the physical body. Heart patients learned exercises to strengthen their aerobic system. Personal clients began to change their eating habits in efforts to return to their ideal weight.

I turned to the gym, the mountains, the bike paths and the pool, child in tow, in my own quest to buff up my body.

In these earlier years, fitness became my religion. My ego had a seat front and center evidenced by my sporting a black bikini at the local swim club.

As I completed my first triathlon, I wanted to shout out to those middle school gym captains who never picked me for their team: "Look at me now!"

Between my job, child rearing and a struggling marriage, I left little room for the spiritual. My moment of awe in the delivery room slipped into a storage unit in a long-forgotten city.

Janice, my friend with whom I could share anything, be totally myself, show up anytime as if I were family, suggested I try yoga.

In her non-judgmental way, she let me know more than once how good yoga would be for me. Into the rooms of *Ashtanga* yoga I entered, to discover the pleasure of elongated muscles, deeply filled lungs and a body working in synchronicity to a new language.

Our teacher invited us to let go of our busy thoughts. She taught us to quiet the chatter in our mind. Slogans like "stay on your own mat" began to make sense.

My ocean breaths represented an hour of vacation in my crazy, busy day. I sopped up every last drop of yoga wisdom like a piece of crusty french bread in a bowl of flavorful bouillabaisse (vegetarian, of course).

Craving more, I began rolling out my mat at home, and my morning practice became a sanctuary for my thoughts. This morning ritual evolved into years of learning and immersion in the yoga world. My vocabulary expanded to include *chakras*, *koshas*, and *bandas*.

The teachings resonated with me deeply.

Integration of body and mind just makes sense. In today's world so much of our health care is segmented into specialties.

Stomach aches? Go to a gastroenterologist.

Chronic headaches? See a neurologist.

Though I'm simplifying and generalizing a bit, my point is that everything is connected.

We are not just a collection of organs and limbs. My baby nurses and my uterus contracts. Hormones travel throughout our body and brain. Emotions regulate our hormones. We are complex beings in need of integrated attention.

I truly appreciated and continue to value the integrated attention of an authentic yoga practice in my own life, and began seeing a need for it in my work with private clients as well.

As my personal training business flourished, I became privy to the life stories of my clients. Appointments were not just about building bulk or running in a race. Some needed strength to cope with a chronic illness. Others wanted to experience the feeling of success in reaching a lifelong goal. I therefore decided to add yoga to my professional toolbox and thus became a registered yoga teacher.

As a practitioner in a diverse religious and secular community, I offer classes in my home yoga studio and travel to other cities to lead programs in yoga, dance, and health.

Many participants have questions about practicing yoga as observant Jews. Some have even asked me to call it something other than yoga when publicizing a workshop.

While toying with the idea of renaming yoga, I fear that we will lose participants who are drawn to the practice for healthy, safe benefits. Wine is used in Judaism to add holiness to a religious ceremony; yet in excess it can also debase one's soul. Similarly, instead of eliminating yoga from the Jewish repertoire, we may instead simply need to sensitize ourselves to its dangers while extracting its gems.

Chew Your Food

One can harvest many jewels from a yoga practice that extends off the mat. One such gem is help in avoiding certain sins we Jews struggle with.

On *Yom Kippur*, we strike our chests during *viduy*, our confessional to G-d for sins we have committed personally or collectively. Particularly difficult are the sins like gluttony—extravagant or wasteful overindulgence in food, drink or wealth—that we commit regularly without awareness.

Here we can learn from those ensconced in the yoga world where much attention is given to mindfulness. Dharma Mittra, known as "the teacher's teacher" and one of the most accomplished yogis in the West, has spent his career teaching yoga in order to serve humanity. His simple yet profound guidelines for the yoga student in his book *Asanas: 608 Yoga Poses* include the following gems:

> "Use discrimination before any action, making sure your actions are honest, respectful, and right.
>
> Maintain a light diet: juices, fruits, salads after 6 p.m. You'll have a good sleep and wake up refreshed. Your stomach must be empty during sleep because that's when the body repairs itself; with food in it the body is occupied with digestion so you wake up more tired than when you went to sleep."

And the grand finale:

> "...If you control your mouth— what you put into it and what comes out of it—you've controlled much of your mind already."

It is commonplace at yoga retreats to minimize waste, recycle paper and plastic, and eat slowly and deliberately. During my stays at Kripalu years ago,

I remember with great appreciation some of these practices.

Bend and stretch, reach for the sky.

It's 6 a.m. and we are already on our yoga mats.

An hour and a half of bodily gyrations wakes me and my appetite.

I make my way to the communal cafeteria and fill my tray with miso, millet, and scrambled tofu.

A large bowl the size of one's cupped hands sits below a sign that instructs us to take no more than a bowlful per meal.

Sitting in the silent dining room, I notice a card propped up on the table in front of me. It states simply "Chew your food."

Gazing around the cavernous hall, I see students pausing before lifting their forks. Private prayers of gratitude float throughout the room.

"Thank you for this food...thank you to those who prepared it, from the growing of the seed, to the planting, harvesting, plucking, and purchasing. What I have in front of me is abundant and I will be satisfied with what I have."

Readers, does any of this sound familiar?

What about the manna?

When the Jews were in the desert for 40 years, G-d prepared, planted and harvested the manna for us to eat. The manna fell from the sky and onto the ground. He instructed us to take only what we needed for that day. This wafer-like food took on the flavor of what we desired, a reference to mindful thought. There was always enough for us.

While my yoga education emphasized the values of moderation, mindfulness, and protection of the world we live in, sadly these values are often neglected in observant Jewish life.

Boundaries are broken as platters multiply at the Shabbos table.

Garbage cans overflow with disposable foil pans and paper products in order to save time on preparation and cleanup.

Half-full plates are scraped into the trash in the kitchens of wedding halls and *bar mitzvah* celebrations.

Meat is consumed in gargantuan portions far beyond the respectable amount needed to honor the Sabbath and *chaggim*, or holidays.

I am often embarrassed by greedy behaviors at the *Kiddush* blessing over wine, following Sabbath prayer.

You know what I'm talking about. The rabbi has not yet said the blessing, and already some congregants are filling their plate with as much *cholent* and as many brownies as will fit on the six-inch diameter plates.

Fork in hand, mouth watering, they wait for the exact nanosecond that the rabbi finishes.

The contents of the plate are then shoved into the mouth and in the blink of an eye, the food has disappeared. Those patient souls at the end of the line stare at the bowls of salad and stew, wondering if there will be any left by the time they reach the ladle.

The people wolfing down their food, taking more than they physically need, preparing and serving quantities beyond reason, are often the same people who frown at yoga.

Learning From Yoga

Perhaps we in the observant Jewish community can glean some lessons from yoga. Lessons such as moderation, mindfulness, and respect for the body might be useful in abolishing the sin of gluttony.

The study of Torah and Talmud are among the most important *mitzvot* in Judaism, and one does not have to delve too deeply to hear about the *yetzer hara*, the evil inclination.

I've often heard guilt-ridden dessert-driven individuals claim, "My *yetzer hara* made me eat it!"

For those not familiar with this phrase, its equivalent is "the devil made me do it." *Yetzer hara* is that gremlin that sits on your shoulder playing devil's advocate when you really, really want to resist temptation.

Mussar helps us learn how to temper our urges.

We must reflect back on our thoughts, speech, and actions—the garments of our souls—in order to examine our behaviors.

The elders of the Hasidic tradition in Orthodox Judaism speak of the animal soul, *nefesh habehamit*, and our Godly soul, *nefesh elokit*.

Our animal soul desires physical pleasures in this world. When we perform a *mitzvah*, or commandment, we introduce our Godly soul into our action, often called *yetzer tov* or "good inclination," and pacify our animal urges. We elevate our action to one which is holy.

For example, blessing our food before we eat it elevates the food and the action of consumption. Because we as humans have free will, we are able to choose our actions. By choosing to elevate our behaviors and thoughts through Godly awareness, we continue to evolve as spiritual beings.

This is a powerful thought. I am not imprisoned by my past actions or thoughts. I am continually renewing myself and choosing my path.

I can choose to live in my animal soul, seeking only physical pleasures and feeding my ego, or I can elevate my life, my purpose, my soul by connecting with something much greater than myself.

I hope that we all have had moments of awe in our lives. Perhaps we were lifted from the mundane while reaching the summit of a mountain, loving another human being, or when giving or witnessing the birth of a child.

The emotions attached to these moments differ greatly from those experienced by the animal soul alone. Buying a new outfit, dining at a fine restaurant, and winning money at a casino are all nice experiences, but not particularly Godly on their own.

And like the concept of opening our vessels in

yoga, once we learn how to quiet our mind and open our physical body, we can use our free choice to consciously choose what we allow to enter—what we open ourselves to.

Yoga acknowledges the connection of body and soul. The word "yoga" itself is derived from a Sanskrit word meaning "to yoke"—we are yoking mind and body. The challenge for Jewish yoga students is to now decide what we let in and what we leave behind.

One way Jews increase their awareness of our G-d-given body is to recite the *Asher Yatzar* prayer after using the bathroom:

> "Blessed are You, HaShem, our
> G-d, King of the Universe, Who
> fashioned man with wisdom
> and created within him many
> openings and many cavities. It is
> obvious and known before Your
> throne of glory that if but one of
> them were to be ruptured or but
> one of them were to be blocked
> it would be impossible to survive
> and to stand before You for
> even one hour. Blessed are You,
> HaShem, who heals all flesh and
> acts wondrously."

One can start this practice by simply saying it every morning, and then progress to reciting it throughout one's day.

Another prayer found in the Sabbath service

beautifully expresses our service to G-d in the physical realm. In this excerpt from the *Nishmat*, our entire body praises G-d:

"The soul of every living being shall bless Your Name, Hashem our G-d, the spirit of all flesh shall always glorify and exalt Your remembrance, our King...

Were our mouth as full of song as the sea, and our tongue as full of joyous song as its multitude of waves, and our lips as full of praise as the breadth of the heavens, and our eyes as brilliant as the sun and the moon, and our hands as outspread as the eagles of the sky and our feet as swift as hinds -- we still could not thank You sufficiently, HaShem our G-d and G-d of our forefathers, and to bless Your Name for even one of the thousand thousand, thousands of thousands and myriad myriads of favors, miracles and wonders that you performed for our ancestors and for us...the organs that you set within us and the spirit and soul that you breathed into our nostrils, and the tongue that you placed in our mouth - all of them

shall thank and bless and praise
and glorify, exalt and revere, be
devoted, sanctify and declare the
sovereignty of Your Name, our
King. For every mouth shall offer
thanks to You; every tongue shall
vow allegiance to You; every
knee shall bend to You; every
erect spine shall prostrate itself
before You; all hearts shall fear
You; and all innermost feelings
and thoughts shall sing praises
to Your name, as it is written: "All
my bones shall say, 'Hashem who
is like You? You save the poor
man from one who is stronger
than he, the poor and destitute
from the one who would rob
him."

My physical practice of yoga and exercise
intermingled with contemplative prayer such as the
Nishmat allows me to draw closer to my Creator and
serve G-d with joy and gratitude.

My workouts are no longer serving my ego in
hopes that I will look terrific in that black bikini.
Don't get me wrong; it's human to want to look
attractive and fit. However, when it becomes our main
focus, we diminish our soul's expression.

A close friend of mine dabbled in online dating,
without much success. As she put it, "I just want to
meet a normal guy, someone I can have an intelligent

conversation with."

Disappointingly, the responses she received bordered on inappropriate. I offered to take a look at her profile and tweak it if needed. The minute I opened her page I saw a beautiful woman displaying serious cleavage. It was impossible not to notice her shapely figure. My friend did not intentionally try to flaunt her shapely body, but the men looking at her profile were drawn to her physical attributes nonetheless. She decided to change her picture in hopes of attracting a man interested in more than her body.

Tempering excessive focus on our physical attributes allows us to keep our egos in check.

Yoga practice on my mat, at the dinner table, and at the *shul Kiddush* allows me to partner with G-d in keeping all of my vessels open.

Seeing my life anew, as a series of connections from prayer to action, is as life-affirming as birthing my child.

9: Sanskrit

Removing Obstacles

"Eka pada rajakapotasana."

There, I said it!

After months of memorizing flash cards, I had painstakingly memorized the Sanskrit names of the half-pigeon pose and so many others that my body knew well.

Despite my resistance to learning this unfamiliar language, I believed it was necessary to advance as a yoga teacher. Didn't my students expect me to announce each pose in its native tongue?

On a later trip to Israel, I was hired to lead a group of seminary students in YogaDance. Yarden, a young, hip dancer with long flexible limbs, flowed through the movements like a graceful gazelle. She had been practicing yoga for years, and was now exploring her Jewish roots at a school nestled in the Judean Hills.

Following the dance workshop, Yarden was eager to invite me to a local yoga class held in a resident's home. Waking early to the bright Israeli sun, I crept out of my bunk to trek up the hills that hauntingly welcomed me.

I can still remember the feast of that morning hike...the unexpected flowers flourishing in the desert, the smell of pure air, and the feeling of full breath in my exercised lungs.

And most memorable, the unspoken whispers of history in those hills.

As I approached the rambling ranch, I saw soon-to-be friends entering the home studio. Women with wrapped scarves on heads and skirts layered over Lululemon leggings suggested I would feel right at home here.

Kissing the *mezuzah* hung on the door post, they entered with mat in hand.

No deities in this yoga studio, I remarked to myself.

Our teacher led us in a perfectly balanced practice, including elements of breath, stretch, strength, and relaxation. Her flowing words described the poses, using the languages of both English and Hebrew. Not one word of Sanskrit was mentioned, and yet I knew exactly what to do.

If yoga is designed to remove obstacles, then this

class succeeded, at least for this student.

Upon returning home to Ohio, I grappled with the language I would use in my own teaching. Sanskrit? English? Hebrew?

I decided to begin referring to the poses in English. I still slip once in a while and throw in a "parsvakonasana" when I can't recall its English equivalent, "extended side angle pose." It now feels awkward, like putting on a six-year-old shirt, wondering if it is still in style.

My rational side renders Sanskrit benign. After all, many of the names are representative of animals and their character traits. Others, like tree pose, have their roots in nature. A closer look reveals names with Hindu origins, such as *Virabadrasana*. This warrior pose refers to Virabhadra, a mythic warrior-sage with one thousand heads. If I want to embody warrior-like characteristics like strength and determination, referring to the pose as "warrior" is more likely going to create that intention.

As a student, I searched my memory each time the teacher called out a pose in Sanskrit. If I could not find the translation in my rudimentary Sanskrit vocabulary, I took my eyes off my own mat and onto another's. Surely the Gumby-like student front and center knew what the teacher was talking about!

Yoga students and teachers alike are allowed to try on these words and see what fits for them. Yoga is not a one-size-fits-all practice. As *Viniyoga* originator Gary Krafstow teaches, the yoga should serve the student; the student does not serve the yoga.

10: Sabbath

Letting The Mud Settle

We yoga teachers like to borrow from each other. The general rule of thumb is that we first reference the source until the principle or practice becomes an organic part of our own teaching.

My wise and wonderful teacher, Linda Oshins, taught us to "sit long enough to let the mud settle." Perhaps she borrowed that slogan from one of her teachers or perhaps it was her own creation. Either way, I think it, teach it and appreciate the process of letting everything, including the mud, settle before entering into any *asana*.

Like mud, life off the mat can get thick and messy, like the week before sending your last child to

sleepaway camp, or the overtime at work prior to a
well-deserved vacation. Once the house is empty or
we've arrived in Bermuda, it is necessary to just sit
and sip in the moment, with a gin and tonic or simply
a chaise longue.

"Letting the mud settle."

It sounds like such a simple, sensible thing. Do
nothing. Rest. No, not by watching three episodes of
reality television, or mindlessly eating a container of
Graeter's raspberry chip ice cream, but by truly just
sitting...with ourselves.

The bookends of a well-balanced yoga class
include a centering or "mud-settling" period at the
start of class and a relaxation period at the end of the
practice, appropriately termed "corpse pose." Without
this structured and designated time for rest, many of
us would wait until we were dead in the ground before
submitting to 10 minutes of non-doing.

By attending yoga classes weekly, I gave myself
permission to indulge in these exquisite slices of
time. I found myself craving corpse pose. Hugger
Mugger's online yoga store was a regular destination
as I ordered yoga props like eye pillows, yoga
blankets, and bolsters, all to help me rest and relax
for a few precious minutes.

Yet the usefulness of my closet full of props paled
in the face of laundry, paperwork and lengthy to-do
lists.

This disease of overdoing was confirmed by the
ayurvedic doctor I sought out for a variety of minor

ailments. After examining my tongue, skin, and the quality of my pulse, he wrote the following on a prescription pad:

> "Savasana (corpse pose) for 20
> minutes daily between the hours
> of 4 and 6 p.m."

Here is the picture he drew for me:

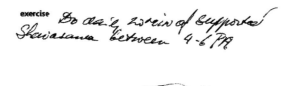

This medication for rest was difficult to swallow.

I had places to go, people to see, things to do.

Enter *Shabbat.*

Yes, I had read about it many times in my prayer book.

G-d rested on the seventh day after He created the Earth.

Okay, that was a long time ago.

Some Jews I knew, including my bearded black-hat brother, kept the Sabbath. But I was not *that* religious, nor did I want to be.

However, with wisdom beyond his years and an unconditional love for me, my big brother simply said to me and my resistant lifestyle, "If you want to be a Reform Jew, know what you are reforming yourself from."

He was right. What exactly was I rejecting? Why was I so open to a practice steeped in Hinduism and so closed to an observance followed by my ancestors and other Jews worldwide?

I have many friends who are well-informed Reform Jews. They have made an educated conscious choice to observe the Sabbath in a way that is authentic to their understanding. I had not learned enough to even make such an informed decision.

In the Meditation chapter, I spoke of my journey towards Sabbath observance as an experience of learning by doing: "*naaseh v' nishmah*. This phrase, "we will do and we will learn," expresses the need to engage so that we may fully understand.

In yoga, we practice poses before fully appreciating their benefit. The poses grow on us, and then one day we are fully planted in downward dog and all effort ceases. We are no longer *doing* the pose, we are *in* the pose. We get it.

Taking on Sabbath begins with details.

Buy the bigger box of candles to commit to the weekly lighting.

Stock up on the Manischewitz Concord grape wine for *Kiddush*.

Tell the teenagers to stay home for Friday night dinner.

Before you know it, the Friday afternoon schedule is cleared to allow time for homemade challah dough to rise.

Time passes. The details become regular rituals, and Friday night begins to blend with Saturday. Before long, we are not only experiencing a day of rest, we become restful.

It's hard to put into words the essence of living a life with a day of rest. It becomes so much more than a restful day once a week. Life takes on a rhythm. Amid the unpredictable chaos of the week, I can count on the gifts of rest and renewal.

What once seemed like restrictions are now blessings. No cell phone glued to my ear. No errands. The laundry room is off limits. My cozy Shabbat chair and stack of books await me.

The feeling is like the comfort of your own familiar yoga mat rolled out on the floor of a lonely hotel room in a faraway city...

Nowhere To Go, Nothing To Do

...or the sigh of relief upon seeing a trail marker after wandering lost for hours.

My husband and I are big hikers.

Every year we strap on thirty-pound backpacks and make our way into the deepest part of the mountains until we find the perfect place to pitch our tent. We look for bubbling brooks, sheltering trees, and a quiet spot devoid of other campers.

It's a lot of work to prepare for such a trip. One has to have the right equipment, proper clothing, and appropriate food. Sometimes it seems like too much effort and we consider forgoing the annual trip.

But we are in it together, and we manage to prepare, pack and strap on the gear. The hike itself holds moments of challenge as well, necessitating a bit of mutual encouragement to continue the climb.

But when we arrive at our long-sought oasis, drop our packs, and hunker down under the stars, it's all worth it.

Nowhere to go, nothing to do. We are simply there to enjoy Creation.

Late at night, lying in our sleeping bags, protected by the walls of our tent, we can feel the quiet around us. Our bodies are so tired from the day's hike. We relax knowing the morning will wake us naturally.

Before we fall asleep, we marvel at how lucky we are to experience this moment...how fortunate we are that we can take this trip into G-d's world and feel such peace.

That's what Shabbat is once you get there.

Yoga on Shabbat

During my yoga teacher training, we were required to practice daily for 30 minutes and record our experience. Pleasure turned into drudgery. Once my training ended, I took a long hiatus before returning to my mat.

Because I teach yoga five days every week, I choose not to practice much on Shabbat. Work is prohibited on the Sabbath unless it's required in order to save lives.

That said, there are times on Shabbat when I go into my home studio, roll out my mat, and practice restorative yoga or breathing in my desire to deepen my focus for the day.

It is said that on Shabbat we are given an extra soul. This extra soul, according to Rashi, a famous medieval Biblical scholar, has an inner and outer purpose.

The outer purpose is an expanded heart, which heightens our senses.

Rafael Moshe Luria in his Chabad.org article "The Additional Shabbat Soul" translated by Simcha Benyosef eloquently explains that the inner purpose "is to help us focus our entire mind on the Almighty. As a result, our ability to feel His Presence is intensified, particularly at the moment of prayers."

He goes on to explain that Shabbat creates space for us to study Torah simply to serve our Creator, putting our ego aside. We forget about material gain, therefore freeing ourselves to reach spiritual heights.

With this intention of clearing my mind and connecting more deeply to this extra soul, I may choose some restorative poses to first allow my body to relax. Often I focus on my breathing while in these poses. The breath for me acts as a bridge from my physical body to my soul.

After preparing my body and mind for relaxation, I move into Jewish meditation, often drawing from the practices highlighted in Rabbi Kaplan's book *Jewish Meditation*. I may work toward visualizing G-d's name or ask a question and listen for the answer.

Some days nothing profound happens. Other days I find myself moved to tears for no reason other than gratitude and connection to something much greater than myself.

Another practice I have come to embrace on *Shabbat* is that of Torah study and reading of Jewish texts.

All week long I am bombarded by news of what is going on in the world, some of which I would rather not know about. Dr. Andrew Weil, an expert in the field of mind-body health, suggests we all take a media vacation from time to time in order to reduce our stress level. Sabbath provides that sanctuary from the barrage of media that is unavoidable during the week.

Often I hear others say that G-d is not there for them; that G-d does not answer their prayers. One does not have to have complete faith in order to try on the idea of a Sabbath.

My rabbi explained to me that when I start to talk to G-d through prayer and *mitzvot*, such as observing the Sabbath, it's as if I am reaching out to a friend I have lost touch with. If I want a relationship with this friend, I need to keep in touch and call her once in a while. In addition, I might think of making time for her in my busy schedule.

Sabbath is a way for me to create space for G-d to

enter. My prayer on this day of rest is not rushed. I don't have another agenda.

These days, my kids are young adults, and as an empty-nester, Sabbath days are often quiet and contemplative. However, Sabbath can bring other gifts, like a Monopoly game with a teenage son who barely has time for his mom during the week. Or visiting with a room full of your children's friends, privy to their deepening thoughts and feelings. Or taking a leisurely walk with a loved one, without the fear of interruption by a cell phone.

Yes, these moments can happen without Shabbat. But when we create space for the sacred, we roll open our mat for the experiences to unfold.

11: The Tree of Yoga

Most Americans associate yoga with physical movements that stretch, strengthen, and relax the body. However, physical yoga—*hatha* yoga—is but one branch of a much larger tree. If we take a look at the other five branches, we see a variety of ways to practice yoga.

And each finds a counterpart in the three pillars of Jewish faith: Torah, meaning study; *avodah*, meaning prayer; and *chesed*, the act of loving kindness.

Devotion to the Divine

Bhakti yoga represents the path of devotion. The focus of this practice is in recognizing the Divine in everyone. Mara Carrico, contributing author to *Yoga Journal*, speaks of Mahatma Gandhi and Martin Luther King, Jr. as examples of individuals who have chosen the path of *bhakti* yoga. They express their devotion, she explains, through their every thought, word, and deed.

Déjà vu? Jews have a devotional path as well.

And through the garments of the soul I described earlier, Jews are to examine their every thought, word, and deed in their interactions with others.

The Study of Sacred Texts

Jnana yoga constitutes the branch of yoga committed to study of scripture and texts in yogic philosophy. In researching the subject of *jnana* yoga, I was interested to see that Kabbalistic scholars were sometimes mentioned in conjunction with Jesuit priests and Benedictine monks as examples of *jnana* yogis.

Though these scholars may all study texts, the content differs vastly. What is important to glean from this reference, however, is that there is clearly a Jewish path to wisdom. One can spend a lifetime studying Torah and Talmud, *Ethics of our Fathers*, Psalms, *mussar*, *Kabbalah* and endless commentary from wise scholars. Even if we intellectually dabble in study of other religions, a Jewish soul remains Jewish and hungers for nourishment from its roots.

How do we decide what our level of belief is if we choose not to study its precepts? Torah cannot be grasped simply by reading the text alone.

Its intricate and often hidden meanings require dialogue, questioning, and often arguing about the text with a partner or teacher.

Unfortunately, many Jews have barely skimmed the surface when they cease their study following *bar mitzvah* or *bat mitzvah*. This is an age when children are finally ready to take on more responsibility as Jews and begin to truly delve into their learning.

As a result, many adults, myself included, are not given the tools necessary to grow in their faith or in knowledge of their Judaism.

Feeling deprived of spiritual strength, many of us have turned to practices outside Judaism. Hebrew, the language of the Torah, is a tongue rich in meaning and beauty. In order to fully appreciate the essence of what the Torah is saying, a student must understand Hebrew. Often the meaning is lost in translation, or the translation is incorrect. Though I have the option of learning Hebrew as an adult, learning it as a child would have served me well, as I struggle today to grasp the meanings in this ancient language.

When my children were in preschool, our neighbor Ernie asked us where we would send them to kindergarten. She taught at the local Jewish day school and just assumed that because we were Jewish, we would consider it.

Our first reaction was to tell her that we had no intention of sending them to the Jewish school. We did not keep kosher or observe *Shabbat*, and we did not see the value in teaching our children Hebrew.

Ernie then asked us, "Will you teach your children calculus when they are in high school?" My husband responded that we most likely would, especially if it were part of the curriculum.

Ernie: "Why will they take calculus?"

Us: "They may need calculus in life."

Ernie: "Don't you think they might need their Judaism as well?"

As we continued our discussion, Ernie asked us what kind of experience we had in "Sunday school," the once- or twice-weekly classes in Jewish studies taken by children after school. We unanimously recalled rather negative experiences.

Not only did we dread attending Sunday morning religious school, we both felt we retained little from our rudimentary education.

Later that week, I found myself in a Jacuzzi at the Jewish Community Center next to a witty, friendly teenager named Talia. After chatting with her, I discovered she was a student at the local Jewish day school. She raved about her experience there, and I could not help but be impressed by her confidence and love of her faith.

When I asked her if she felt isolated from the rest of the world by restricting herself to a Jewish day school, she claimed, "On the contrary. I know who I am and where I came from. I can talk to anyone now with confidence because I am clear in my beliefs."

In some strange way, I believed that meeting Talia was not just coincidence. Nevertheless, my husband and I were not likely to send our children to such a school when we ourselves were barely engaged in our own Jewish practice.

And then, when we had just about put the idea out of our heads, we were informed that our street had been redistricted and our daughter would not be attending the local kindergarten with all of her friends. Instead, she would be bused to another school quite a distance away.

So in an unexpected twist of events, we decided to send her to the Jewish day school, just for a trial period. After all, it was just kindergarten.

Our daughter thrived in day school, thus prompting us to send our son as well. Our children began teaching us the beauty of our heritage. We never looked back.

We are commanded to teach our children Torah. That can be a tall order if we ourselves lack the knowledge or faith necessary to pass on the torch of Jewish knowledge.

As a nurse in the ICU, I was privy to others' innermost prayers and thoughts regarding faith.

I remember a young adult, Paul, who at age 31 was shot in the neck by an angry driver on the Los Angeles freeway.

Paul had competed professionally in tennis, and now his career and his passion was severed along with his spinal cord. Left a quadriplegic, he harbored a large dose of anger toward the world. When the anger subsided, he was left with depression. Not a man of faith, he did not have the tools of prayer or faith to lift the sadness.

Pilar, a beautiful dark-haired 18-year-old girl from Mexico, was visiting California on vacation when she took a ride on a motorcycle.

After a tragic accident, Pilar, who had not been wearing a helmet, lay in a coma in the hospital in which I worked.

As her primary nurse, I came to know her family, who diligently took turns at her bedside day after day. How does a parent cope with such a tragedy?

I can still feel today, 26 years later, the faith and love that flowed from this family, toward their little girl, the staff and to their G-d. As someone longing for such strong ties to G-d, I envied their faith. I marveled at how they could show up every day with such hope, such love in their hearts.

We all have free choice: to believe or not to believe. To learn or not to learn. If we are lucky enough to believe, or willing enough to learn and grow our belief, the journey through life's great challenges is blanketed with comfort.

Selfless Service

Karma yoga, often referred to as selfless service to others, is extremely compatible with Jewish thought and practice. In fact, it is one concept that is embraced by all sects of Judaism.

I look back with fond memories of the myriad volunteer opportunities I had while growing up in the Reform movement. From serving food at the soup kitchens to delivering food for Meals on Wheels, not a week went by without our community helping someone in need.

Yogis believe that our past actions shape our present experience. Judaism, a religion of action, emphasizes the deeds we do in this world. Though we may not receive rewards in this life, G-d takes notice of all we do and rewards us accordingly in *Olam Haba*, the world to come.

We will then be judged not in comparison to each other, but whether we lived up to our own potential. We all have a responsibility to emulate kindness toward others through *chesed*, acts of loving kindness, and to help those less fortunate.

Unfortunately, though we as Jews share the precept of *chesed*, many of us are quick to judge Jews who practice in ways different from our own.

We all too often label others based on how they look or which synagogue they attend. Our past does shape who we are today, and all of us have differing experiences that alter the lens through which we see our world.

As a blended family, my husband and I have four very different children. They have all chosen widely different ways to express their Judaism. One child studies in a yeshiva and *davens*, or prays, three times a day in a formal setting.

Another child spent two years in the Peace Corps, teaching a poor African community how to improve its health.

Who are we to say what is more valued in G-d's

eyes? He is the only judge. Service to others is selfless if we are humbled through the process.

This global principle of spreading "good karma" links us all together, Jews and those of other faiths as well.

We stand before G-d always, and if we conduct ourselves with that awareness, we will show acts of loving kindness to all.

Desire and the Divine

Tantra yoga focuses on bringing the sacred into sexuality. As I attended *ashrams* and yoga retreats, we were often asked to adhere to *brachmacharya*, loosely translated as celibacy.

Our teachers felt that if we became involved in new relationships of a sexual nature, our energy would be dispersed and our focus on furthering our study of yoga would be diminished.

In addition, we had an unspoken respect for each other, manifested by giving fellow participants space to work on themselves.

Intimate relationships between teacher and student were frowned upon, though scandals emerged not infrequently as human temptation overcame even the most sincere of practitioners.

These developments were not surprising; when we open up our bodies through various poses and unleash the *chakras*, the wheels of energy throughout our bodies, we may experience a desire to connect physically with another.

In Judaism, we also embrace the sacred in our sexuality.

As I discussed in the chapter on Meditation, the laws of *taharat hamishpacha*, or family purity, provide boundaries for Jews to sanctify and protect the intimate, sacred connection with our *basherte*, our soulmate.

Though many discard this practice as antiquated or degrading to women, these laws are intricate and require study and practice in order to fully understand and appreciate their merit and beauty.

We are all too aware of the infidelity, divorce, and discontent in an unhealthy proportion of marriages today. Couples often speak of boredom and apathy in their relationship after years of predictable exchanges with each other.

Can you as a reader remember the excitement of dating? The feeling of falling in love? Wondering what you would do together, what you would wear, when you would see each other next?

Recently I was talking with a young woman who was engaged to be married. She waited impatiently for her wedding day to arrive.

I wanted to say to her, "Enjoy this time! The mystery in your relationship is something to savor."

Safety, stability and comfort are universal needs. Strong marriages meet these needs. However, we as humans also have needs for renewal, creativity and intrigue. The laws of family purity provide a healthy balance in marriages for these needs to be met.

Psychologists who counsel couples in matters of sexual difficulties will often suggest periods of enforced separation in order to introduce the intrigue and excitement back into the marriage. This technique has been found to be extremely effective in recreating intimacy in marriage.

We as Jews have been given this gift that begins during the dating period. Potential couples refrain from physical touch in order to keep their perspectives unclouded.

Just as yoga students provide a respectful boundary for each other by restricting their physical involvement, so too a dating couple keeps this boundary to focus on attributes and character traits essential to a lasting relationship.

Physical intimacy begins after the wedding, thus introducing a connection that is protected and holy.

I remember a lecture I attended by Dr. Lisa Aiken, a clinical psychologist and international speaker.

She discussed two scenarios of marriage. In one, the husband and wife are connected to each other in a linear fashion. In the second, a triangle exists with G-d at the top of the triangle, thus making the relationship stronger.

If we look at the first marriage, Adam and Eve were created from one body. In a Jewish marriage, the two souls are merged and husband and wife are brought together as one.

The notion of refraining from physical contact prior to marriage, known as *shomer negiah*, may sound utterly ridiculous to an outsider.

However, we need only look at the statistics. The University of Chicago's 1994 *National Health and Social Life Survey* reported a strong connection between premarital intimacy and a higher risk of divorce, as have other, even more recent, academic and governmental studies.

When something is valuable, we want to protect it.

We keep our most important papers and family heirlooms safe in a vault.

Is it so far-fetched to want to keep our relationship with our life partner safe as well?

What boundaries do we provide to safeguard the intimacy of our marriages?

These Jewish laws are not just for the Orthodox. They are available to all Jews, no matter their level of observance.

Rituals Across Generations

Unfortunately, our need to place ourselves in a box or wear a label that identifies just what type of Jew we are may close the door to a myriad of meaningful rituals. The beauty of ritual is felt not only in its performance, but in our commitment to passing on its holiness to future generations.

My great-grandmother used the *mikvah*. She sent her daughter to America to save her from Nazi persecution.

My grandmother escaped the gas chambers of

Auschwitz, leaving behind her entire family and many of their traditions. Yet she still made the homemade egg noodles cooked slowly in milk and sugar, just like her mother made for her.

Sometimes in the middle of a sentence, she would switch tongues, and out would come a torrent of Yiddish that only my mother could understand.

And one night while tucking me into bed, Grandma Jean sang a song to me, in her fragile, creaky voice:

"Bei mir bistu shein, please let me explain, bei mir bistu shein, that means you're grand…"

Arriving in a new country with only a few coins in her pocket and some old jewelry sewn into her coat, she and her new husband soon abandoned Shabbat, working assiduously instead to make ends meet. In an effort to assimilate into the new culture, traditions such as *mikvah* were discarded.

By the time my mother became an adult and married, her family's practices of Shabbat, *mikvah* and *kashrut* had faded along with the recipe for homemade egg noodles.

My mom tried to recreate that sweet, comforting dish, but it never tasted quite the same. In my mother's later years, beyond the time a woman might use the *mikvah*, she returned to the roots of her upbringing and began to study Torah.

Bits of ritual seeped into her home, and connected her to her past. She informed her friends and children of her lifestyle change, kashered the kitchen, and learned the rudiments of the *Shabbos* service.

And then she decided to reclaim her birthright to experience *mikvah*. She shared the deep emotions that this brought forth with a dear friend, who was moved to write this essay honoring her experience:

> Taking The Plunge
>
> "She decided that the time had come to do the mikvah.
>
> Worrying that she wasn't religious enough, knowledgeable enough, she began to read about the mysterious, mystical waters of taharas michpocha, and finally her appointment to immerse was at hand.
>
> It was not, after all, a totally foreign concept, for she vaguely remembers that both her grandmother and mother had gone to the mikvah and, she was but picking up where they left off, continuing the chain of Jewish family tradition.
>
> As she sinks into the warm waters, she feels peaceful and pure, proud and grateful, for now she belongs to the group and has fulfilled the commandment of Hashem.

She reads the inspiring
prayer posted by the waters
by the gentle and patient
Mrs. Markvocik, the mikvah
lady. Finding so much that is
meaningful to her in that prayer,
she begins to weep, and then to
sob. If only my mother were alive
to see me now. She immerses
once, twice, three times, and
wonders if she'll drown from
crying under water.

Then it is over. Mrs. Markovic
envelops her in a hug, and she
races to the private dressing
room to be alone. Her husband
and children are proud.

So is her mother."

On my most recent visit to my daughter's home, as I was rocking my granddaughter to sleep, I found myself singing a song that had been hiding in a crevice of my mind.

"Bei mir bistu shein, please let me explain, bei mir bistu shein, that means you're grand...".

The Contemplative Path

Raja yoga embraces the eight limbs of yoga outlined by yogic scholar Patanjali in the *Yoga Sutra*, the foundational text of *raja* yoga. The principles embodied in the *Yoga Sutra* lead the practitioner along a path of contemplation and meditation. We'll explore these more in the next chapters.

For now, let me just say that in my study of the principles of *raja* yoga I could not help but compare these observances with those found in our Torah.

For those students of yoga seeking such a contemplative path, it is enlightening to know that we as Jews can practice these principles without leaving our own sacred texts and rituals.

Further, we may have a clearer path to such elevated states if we remove the obstacles that block our soul's connection with G-d. Such forces, often referred to as *klipot*, or shells, block the light of G-d from entering our surroundings and our mind. Through Torah study, we will find the blueprint for character refinement.

But, study is not enough. We then need to have the discipline to turn our learning into action.

12: The Yamas

Examination of *raja* yoga's first limb, the five *yamas*, or ethical rules, and how they are practiced by yogis throughout the world gives us as Jews more effective ways to adhere to our own commandments.

Non-Violence

The first of the five behaviors outlined in the *yamas* is *ahimsa*, or non-violence. *Ahimsa* represents more than the absence of violence. Here we are instructed not only to refrain from cruelty to any living creature, but in addition to speak and act with kindness and thoughtfulness toward others, including ourselves.

As part of my 500-hour Registered Yoga Teacher training, our curriculum included the study of nonviolent communication. To this day I am incredibly grateful to my teacher Marcia Miller for teaching me about respectful boundaries for myself.

As a caretaker, I often stepped over my own needs in order to people-please. Once I learned how to express my own feelings and needs, I was then able to empathize with others in a healthy way. My training in this form of compassionate communication provided the tools necessary to clear out anger from my repertoire of reactions.

My son-in-law Jon studies in a *yeshiva* in New York, preparing to become a rabbi. Though he has never entered a yoga studio in his life, he practices *ahimsa* daily. While driving on the freeways of the city, he uses the stops at the toll booths to spread kindness to complete strangers. As he is paying his toll, he makes a point to ask the collector how his or her day is going.

Such a small gesture, you may say, but I have witnessed the smiles of those he treats with humanness. We can change someone's day just by acknowledging that they exist.

In an ongoing effort to engage in Torah learning, my husband and I studied the text "*Iggeres Ha Ramban*" or "The Ramban's Letter."

This letter was written by a great Torah scholar to his son, and expounds upon the importance of controlling one's anger. The ultimate goal is to humble oneself with the awareness that he or she is standing before G-d always.

He instructs, "Get into the habit of always speaking calmly to everyone. This will prevent you from anger, a serious character flaw which causes people to sin."

In an effort to turn this Torah study into action, I now need to discipline myself toward daily reflection on this valuable text. It may take a lifetime of effort to eliminate anger from my thoughts, speech and actions. But regular practice and focus on this character trait will create change toward a peaceful heart.

The story of Rabbi Akiva illustrates this point. As a laborer and shepherd, forty-year-old Akiva had little knowledge of Torah. While gazing at a trickle of water, he noticed the effect the dripping had on the rock below it. Through the slow steady drop of water, a hole had been carved. He then surmised that if soft water could penetrate hard stone, so too could words of Torah enter his forty-year-old heart. And so he began the process of Torah study, and became a revered scholar, passing on his teachings to over 24,000 students in his time.

I have found a teacher of this principle in my stepdaughter, Arielle. In the 13 years I have known her, I have never heard her yell or raise her voice. She thinks deeply before speaking, and displays honor to her father and me at all times. Her *middot*, or character traits, have been formed by living an ethical life, practicing guarded speech, and in service to others.

By committing ourselves to refinement of our

character flaws, we too can remove anger from our hearts.

Another area of potential violence is in our consumption of food.

A majority of yogis throughout the world have chosen to adopt vegetarianism in order to minimize violence toward animals.

The Jewish practice of *kashrut* is supposed to limit cruelty toward the animals we consume for food. Included in the laws of *shehita*, or ritual slaughter, are instructions to show respect and compassion by killing the animal with the least amount of pain possible.

There is a growing body of Jews who are concerned not only with how animals are slaughtered for consumption, but also with how they are raised.

One will find arguments for and against pairing ethical practice with *halacha*, the Jewish body of religious laws. I am suggesting that we as Jews make ourselves aware of the issues and make informed choices about the food we are eating.

For some, practicing nonviolence may mean adopting a vegan or vegetarian diet. For others, choosing to buy pastured meat that has been raised ethically is a step toward more conscious eating. And for yet others, it may be as simple as consuming fewer animal products.

In a religion that advocates humane treatment for all and sanctity for life, it behooves us to look at how the production of food, whether animal or vegetable, has changed in our world today.

After all, we as humans have the ability to decipher what heals and what hurts. In choosing to control and select what we put into our bodies, we tame the animal in all of us.

Speaking Truth

The second *yama* in *raja* yoga is *satya*, or speaking the truth.

Yogis are taught to examine their words before speaking, and to speak truthfully unless doing so would harm another.

Often silence is practiced as a way to reflect rather than react to what someone else is saying. Learning how to sit with emotion, especially when it's uncomfortable, is a practice that fosters patience, tolerance, and truth.

In Judaism, truthful speech is also emphasized. *Lashon hora*, translated as "evil tongue", is often used to describe gossip. One who engages in gossip is committing a grave sin. Our words enter the world and are carried and spread to places we cannot reach. Listening to gossip is also considered a sin. Embarking on a path to practice guarding one's tongue and ears is a spiritual practice, and not an easy one. Distancing ourselves from those who speak *lashon hora* is a way to diminish untruths which would otherwise be released into our world.

Truthfulness is nourished when we realize before Whom we are standing. Whether tiptoeing through a child's room to uncover secrets or cheating on our taxes, it is all lying in the face of G-d.

Those of us with a healthy conscience know quite well the feeling that permeates our insides when we entertain mistruths.

Like putting the fork down when we are pleasantly full, we can cultivate a practice of telling the truth to ourselves and to others. When I was a young girl, my mother loved to take me shopping for new clothes each season. Squealing with excitement, we rode the escalator in Kaufmann's to the dress department. Selecting a wardrobe that exceeded the clothing budget, out of her pocket slid some cash my mother had kept hidden for moments such as these.

Half of the bill would then be placed on the credit card, the other half paid by her secret stash. My father would never find out how much we really spent on our glorious shopping spree.

I never thought much about these closet transactions until I became an adult and repeated this pattern. The big brown bag contained a large dose of guilt along with my store-bought items.

Little white lies were masked as excuses when reporting my purchases to my husband.

"It was such a great sale...I bought it a long time ago....my mom sent me some spending money."

I carried the irrational fear that my husband would somehow be angry with me.

At times the uneasy feelings created by the guilt and lies prevented me from shopping at all.

Little white lies seeped into other corners of my life as well, serving as protective armor from the reactions of others.

I wanted so much to rid myself of this unspoken fear that had taken up residence in my gut.

And then one day I was sitting in a *shiur*, a Torah lesson, regarding the six constant *mitzvot*, or commandments. The Torah commands us to perform 613 *mitzvot*, but, since it is impossible for any one Jew to perform all of them, our Sages suggest that we all observe six *mitzvot* at all times.

One of these commandments is to fear G-d, as quoted in the Torah reading Devarim 10:20, "Hashem, your G-d, you shall fear."

However, the next constant *mitzvah* is love of G-d.

In combining fear and love, we reach a different translation: that of awe.

The more we draw closer to G-d the more we are in awe of G-d's power and greatness, and the more we feel the reciprocal love between us and our Creator.

The rabbi went on to explain that this fear or awe of G-d is not meant to paralyze us but instead to draw us closer to G-d. As I continued to absorb the teaching, I realized I was lacking in *emunah*, in the belief in G-d's constant presence in my life. Placing my fear in others and hiding behind lies negated my faith in G-d's protection.

I decided to begin a practice of *yirat Hashem*, the practice of speaking truthful words and thinking truthful thoughts. This Torah learning permeated even the hidden pockets of fear I had held since childhood, and my ongoing *avodah*, or work, on this constant *mitzvah* carries me through the struggle.

Non-Stealing

Asteya, or non-stealing, is the third *yama* in yogic philosophy.

I am indebted to my yoga teachers who broadened this principle for us beyond the simple interpretation.

Not only does *asteya* mean to refrain from taking an object that is not ours; it also extends to mindfulness of another's time and space.

Talking too much steals time for others to share and robs us of silent spaces.

Interrupting someone can rob them of their thought process.

Beginning and ending a class on time is another way to implement the practice of non-stealing.

Judaism has a lot to say about stealing.

The Jewish court, or *Beit Din*, assigns punishments for this sin. If a burglar sneaks into a home and takes some of its contents, his penalty is twice the amount of a robber who steals openly, in public, even at gunpoint.

The rationale is that the burglar who commits the crime secretly only fears the person from whom he steals. The robber who steals publicly has no more fear of G-d than he does of people.

Abstinence

Brachmacharya, often thought of as abstinence from sexual activity, is the fourth *yama*.

Here again, yogic and Jewish philosophy are synchronized.

As the *tantra* yoga discussion pointed out, harnessing our sexual energy in certain situations allows us to elevate ourselves spiritually and cultivate safe relationships with others.

In some Jewish circles, married couples choose to refrain from physical contact with members of the opposite sex. Instead of giving my best friend's husband a hug when greeting him, I may choose to acknowledge his presence with a friendly "hello."

I found this practice to be quite difficult at the start as I am a naturally demonstrative person. Over time, I came to appreciate the respect my husband and I gave each other by restricting our physical contact with others. Interactions with other men also felt safer and less flirtatious with my invisible attitude of respectful restraint.

These practices have created healthy boundaries for me in working with male students in the yoga world. Though I may touch a client if necessary to correct an unsafe posture, or to help a pose emerge, it is done with respect and only when truly necessary. My intention to maintain professional and personal space is honored.

Non-Attachment

The fifth and final *yama* is known as *aparigraha*, meaning non-attachment.

This requires releasing the desire to take more than one needs.

Hoarding or collecting material objects represents a lack of faith in G-d's ability to provide for us.

I recall an incident in my teacher training that shook up quite a few of the students. During a weekend workshop, it is typical for each student to "claim" their space, placing their mat and other props in a spot that feels right for them. Each day the student naturally gravitates to the same spot, with an unwritten message of ownership.

One morning, after nesting into our personal spaces, our teacher instructed us to get up and move to a different place in the room. Those pupils who always chose the front row were scoffing as they begrudgingly stomped to the back. As we centered that morning, the silence felt noisy.

"You don't own the space that you choose. Don't get too attached to it," our teacher remarked. We then reflected upon our own tattered security blankets, fringed from overuse.

Were we ready to let go of objects used for status, comfort, or pride?

Jews are also taught to take only what is needed.

When the Jews wandered the desert, G-d sent food to them in the form of manna. If individuals took more than they were able to consume, the remaining manna rotted.

The message? Trust that G-d will provide for us daily.

Today, we are instructed to give 10% of our income to charity without greed.

Because our prosperity is a gift from G-d, all of our money does not belong to us. By giving back to those in need with an open heart, we are trusting that we will have what we need.

How we give is also fundamental. A solicitor ringing our doorbell does not mean that he or she is the one in need. The homeowner, comfortable behind sealed windows and doors and a full refrigerator may be the one with a need—the need to give.

My son is blessed to have a friend for life.

At the age of nine, Alex surfed into my son's life and they have been riding waves since.

Out of the water, their paths have taken them in different directions. Both carry strong internal Jewish identities, yet the way they express their faith varies greatly.

Recently I was able to catch up with Alex and *kvell*, or rejoice, as I discovered the *mensch*, the admirable man he had become. In particular, he shared with me the experience of sorting out his childhood bedroom.

His mom had asked him to weed through the *tchotchkes* and decide what was worth saving. As he looked at the plethora of swimming trophies, ribbons, and plaques on his bookshelf, he realized that he no longer needed physical proof of his accomplishments. He modestly claimed, "All of those races are inside of me."

And with that he discarded every last memento that had praised his skills as the fastest captain of the high school swim team.

Wow... Twenty years old and he has already grasped a concept most of us are still struggling with as adults.

13: The Niyamas

The *niyamas* form the second limb of yoga. Like *yamas*, the five *niyamas*, personal observances that reflect our internal feelings about ourselves, may also offer insights with meaning for us as Jews.

Purity

Sauca, the first *niyama*, means purity or cleanliness. Yogis cleanse their inner body through *asana*, physical yoga, and *pranayama*, breath practice. For example, a yogi might think of a twisting pose as analogous to wringing out a towel. Breath practices such as *nali*, the rolling of the stomach, or *kabhabalabahti*, breath of fire, aim to detoxify the body.

Anyone who has taken a yoga class knows well the

feeling of openness that stretching and breathing can bring.

Setting aside an hour or so to practice allows the participant not just to refresh the body, but also to attend to clearing out the cobwebs of the mind. In a world of cluttered rooms and beeping devices, the gift of a spacious technology-free yoga room is incredibly inviting.

In my yoga classes, held in what used to be my lonely living room, the goal is not necessarily to move deeper into a physical pose, but to make space in the mind for fresh thoughts.

Emotions such as anger, greed, and the more common self-criticism are discarded, making room for acceptance and joy. Physical yoga was first created to promote comfort in the body so that the yogi could sit freely while quieting the mind. Physical pain can be a great obstacle to spiritual enlightenment.

It might benefit those of us who struggle with prayer to prepare for such an ethereal encounter with physical yoga, breath work, or exercise.

One client of mine often exclaims after her workout, "I can feel the blood coursing through my body!". Approaching G-d with the awareness of life allows us to serve G-d with joy and vitality.

When our children are young, we encourage them to run, play, and "get out their aggression" on the playground. We know exercise is good for them, and we try our best to feed them nourishing food. Pregnant women tend to follow their doctor's instructions and are careful to eat healthy foods so that their baby will thrive.

So why is it that as adults, we abandon such healthful practices and substitute hours of Torah study, work obligations, and prayer?

Obviously these *mitzvot* are important, but what happened to the *mitzvah* of caring for our bodies, the vessels that we have been given by G-d?

My nephews are studying in *yeshiva*, and have been for several years. They tell me that once a week they are allotted barely an hour to play basketball.

Once married, there is even less time devoted to fitness. Meals often involve large quantities of food with little attention to health. Plates served at *smachot*, or celebrations, overflow with larger than life portions of meat, kugel, and potatoes. Salty, fatty food is washed down with liters of soda that have multiplied throughout the social hall.

I appreciate the notion of elevating a holiday or special occasion with a lovely meal.

But why is such excess necessary? And why do we feel we are rewarding our children when we give them non-foods like soda and candy?

It is not enough to say *tehillim,* psalms for someone who is ill, for someone with heart disease or diabetes.

Just as the highest form of *tzedakah* is giving people jobs that empower them to earn their own income, let's empower others with good health by encouraging proper care of the body. In this way, we can reduce illness and disease, honoring the *mitzvah* of *pikuach nefesh*, saving a life.

Contentment

Santosa, or contentment, is the second *niyama*. The Dalai Lama expresses *santosa* perfectly in the following quotation:

> "When you are discontent,
> you always want more, more,
> more. Your desire can never be
> satisfied. But when you practice
> contentment, you can say to
> yourself, 'Oh yes - I already have
> everything that I really need.'"

We have all met people who believe that happiness comes once a goal is achieved.

"Once I land that prestigious account, I will be happy. If I just push a little more and work harder, then I will have enough money to feel satisfied."

Spending time with such individuals is exhausting. These George Jetsons of the world are running on a continuously moving treadmill, to a destination that will forever elude them.

Santosa is also translated as modesty.

As a yoga teacher, I am expected to exercise modesty through a variety of vehicles. Acknowledging that I too am a student keeps my ego in check. Teaching students to listen to their internal cues when exploring the depth of a pose is a way to emphasize modesty. The joy in a pose is not in the end result but in the exploration. Being able to put my leg over my head will not necessarily make me more enlightened.

A colleague and I attended a workshop given by a yoga celebrity. Though we gratefully tucked away teaching gems from such an experienced and knowledgeable mentor, we did not enjoy the overlay of show that came with his visit.

Students arrived sporting makeup, perfume and lots of attitude. Neck muscles bulged and toes clenched the mat as they held poses far past their comfort zone.

Was yoga to be a new sport in the upcoming summer Olympics?

I was happy to return to my hometown teacher, with her modest t-shirt and graying hair.

Turning to Jewish thought, modesty and inner happiness temper unhealthy competition.

A common prayer recited by some three times a day is the *Ashrei*, a psalm that begins:

> "Happy are those who dwell in
> Your house..."

A passage found in the middle of the prayer states, "You open Your hand, and satisfy the desire of every living thing."

Though acknowledging this is not always an easy task, we are to hold deeply the belief that everything G-d does is good and that G-d gives us all that we need.

Modesty is a concept that has been misinterpreted by many in Jewish circles. Disagreements among sects regarding appearance have caused violence far beyond finger pointing.

I am greatly saddened by the divisions born out of judgment or fear of what might look different compared to one's own custom.

And yet I have been the bearer of such judgment. I admit it.

In years prior to any serious Jewish study, I gawked at certain groups with critical eyes, wondering why in the world they would wear such dark heavy clothing in the middle of the summer. I felt pity for women who "had" to cover their hair and worried that their rights to freedom were being violated. And as an observant Jew, I have shrieked silently while gazing at cleavage I secretly wished to cover.

This I am not proud of.

I did not fully grasp the concept of modesty until I was asked to explain to an old friend why I began covering my hair.

She and I had been quite close until the learning I soaked up turned into action. She felt morally violated by my head covering and what it represented to her. This division in our friendship helped me to further define my religious beliefs and explain my feelings in a way that fortunately was non-threatening to her.

As I shared with her, in our prayer *Ashrei* we

express the belief that happiness arises as we become closer to our Creator. As we grow in awareness of G-d dwelling inside of us, we connect to the ever-present source of happiness.

My Jewish learning and subsequent action led me to desire more closeness. The covering of my hair was a constant reminder that I was standing before G-d and carrying out G-d's *mitzvot*.

My change in dress provided a way for me to express my modesty and strengthen my internal attributes. With my little black bikini in the Goodwill bag, body parts once exposed were now off limits to the rest of the world.

Each person has free will to explore the level of modesty that protects his or her soul. Respecting others' outward expression without judgment is essential to the health of Judaism.

Tapas

Contentment, *santosa*, is balanced by *tapas*, the third *niyama*. *Tapas* literally means heating the body in order to cleanse it.

Tapas practices unfold through exercise, breath practice, healthy eating, and *asana*, to name a few. Working on *tapas* may appear to contradict *santosa* as a student creates more fire in their practice. Yet it is necessary to move out of one's comfort zone at times to establish a discipline of committed practice and to test one's limits.

I remember vividly the first time I completed

a handstand as an adult. Etched in my brain was a blueprint of instructions: Place your hands on the mat a few inches away from the wall, step back into downward dog, bring one foot forward onto the mat, discard the fear and doubt, kick up with the back leg, let the front leg follow.

Watching the will of other students as they pushed through resistance and overcame their fear of inverting motivated me to finally attempt this physically demanding pose.

Hands on mat, stepping back to downward dog, ready to swing my back leg up toward the protective wall in front of me...I felt anything but protected.

Fear clutched my heart.

"I don't have to prove anything to anyone. If I never do a handstand, I will be just fine."

As if my teacher heard my inner discussion, she stopped the class and said to me in her firm yet reassuring voice, "Shelly, just kick up and do it. You are strong enough. I know you can do it."

With all eyes on me, my fear and I kicked that back leg up to the wall, the other leg came soaring up to meet it, and I found myself upside down, strong and fearless.

Yeah, baby!!!

That's *tapas*. It wasn't about my ego. It wasn't about pleasing my fellow students or obeying my teacher. It was about pushing through my resistance, letting go of the familiar, comfortable place I knew, and working really hard to get to the next level.

I have been rewarded time and again since then with the ease of a handstand: the feeling of floating up to a place of calm strength and confidence.

But more than that, *tapas* brings us the will to move past resistance. *Tapas* keeps us from getting too comfortable with where we are, and propels us to renew our goals. Gandhi so beautifully expressed the need to continuously evolve with his words, "Be the change you wish to see in the world."

Jewish practice also contains *tapas* in ritual and in Torah learning. When we think we have arrived and become set in our ways, we halt our growth and close off our evolving relationship with our Creator. It is important to notice when our faith practice becomes rote. Are we so wise as to say we have arrived?

One practice that may help us to create a bit of fire in our religious lives is to honor our Hebrew birthday each year.

Sites like Chabad.org will calculate your Hebrew birthday, based on the lunar calendar, when you plug in the date and time of your secular birthday, based on the solar calendar.

In recognizing this day, we are thanking G-d for another year of growth and life.

Following the suggestion of another teacher, I have begun to celebrate my Hebrew birthday with a *farbrengen*, a party.

With pitchers of Shelly's famous sangria and a cream-cheese frosted carrot cake crafted by my dear friend Janet, students, friends, and family are all invited to celebrate.

Between the singing, dancing, and schmoozing, words of Torah are spoken. With the support of community, I share my own struggles of faith and commit to another year of growth, biting off a morsel at a time.

In being the change we wish to create, we all work on ourselves and build the Temple to come, one brick at a time.

The physical practice of *tapas* may naturally lead us to a spiritual wellspring.

Our son Daniel has the gift of merging the physical with the spiritual in his everyday life. With an incredible zeal for life, he replenishes his energy regularly through both Torah learning and physical fitness. He has spent much of his young life honing his athletic skills in the sport of the season, from football and basketball to baseball. By far the sport that surpasses them all is surfing.

Show up.

Wade in and get your feet wet.

Move through the choppy, bitingly cold water and plunge in, face and all.

Paddle out to where the waves form, searching for the perfect wave.

Leap onto the board.

Time to ride! Gliding over the shiny, slick surface, rider and wave unite.

It's quiet out there.

And just when you think you are in control, a huge unexpected wave plunges you into the deep dark void.

G-d is running the show.

And within seconds you are back on the shore, shaken up but safe.

Self-Study

Svadhyaya, or the study of one's self, represents the fourth *niyama* of yoga. *Tapas* prepares the physical body for such inquiry.

Setting time aside to reflect on what is working and what still needs attention is necessary to begin this study.

An example of this process is found in the centering portion of a yoga class. We often begin by sitting and observing what is present. How am I feeling today? What am I needing from my practice?

More specifically, we may notice the effects of our previous behaviors. Staying up late watching reruns of "Saturday Night Live" may have left us feeling tired. Drinking two cups of coffee has caused us to feel jittery.

Once we can take the time to observe and then notice the connection between our past behaviors and current state, we can then make a choice to change our course or stay in our discomfort.

At first our observation may simply lead us to basic physical changes.

My hips are tight; I am going to sit on a cushion to

feel greater ease.

Noticing the breath may take us a step deeper. My breath is shallow and short. I will try taking deeper, slower breaths. The breath can bridge the space between the physical and the emotional.

Now that I am breathing, I can invite my mind to be present.

Here comes the good stuff.

I can now ask "What am I needing? What is working?" And perhaps even deeper, "What is my purpose today? Why am I here?".

One exercise I like to offer my clients is based on a favorite quote from author and poet Annie Dillard, who points out in her book *The Writing Life* that "How we spend our days is how we spend our lives."

Students are asked to write on one side of a sheet of paper how they spend their days, listing specifically the activities that occupy the majority of their time.

On the other side of the paper they then write down their most important values. If struggling to identify what these values are, one can ask the rather morbid but thought-provoking question: "What would I want my obituary to say?"

MY VALUES	MY ACTIVITIES
1. My health	1. Working 50 hours/week
2. Family	2. Watching TV
3. Time for leisure	3. Cleaning up after family
4. Service to others	4. Answering emails
	5. Volunteering at food bank

We then compare the two lists and evaluate the degree to which our daily activities reflect our values.

After an honest account, this individual might discover that some of her most important values are not being met. She may decide then to restructure her schedule to allow for exercise, some leisure time, and quality hours with family.

Though this exercise may appear simplistic and overly rational, many of us fail to take time to evaluate our own lives. Yet we are quite good at pointing out others' faults, especially those we love the most.

Be the change...by starting with ourselves.

Does Judaism have its own self-study? Yes. *Cheshbon hanefesh*, an accounting of the soul and of our *middot*, our character traits, is such a practice. We don't need yoga philosophy to perfect ourselves; we have our own approach, steeped in Torah.

In his book *Cheshbon ha-Nefesh*, Rabbi Menachem Mendel, an enlightened scholar of the late 1700s whose mission was to reeducate Jews for life in modern society, guides the reader through the *middot*. He and other scholars illuminate a variety of these traits:

The Middot: Our Character Traits

      ৵ equanimity   ৵ calmness

      ৵ patience   ৵ truth

      ৵ order   ৵ separation

      ৵ decisiveness   ৵ temperance

      ৵ cleanliness   ৵ deliberation

      ৵ humility   ৵ gratitude

      ৵ righteousness   ৵ modesty

      ৵ frugality   ৵ trust

      ৵ zeal   ৵ generosity

      ৵ silence

Jews are instructed to examine their behaviors, including thoughts, speech and actions, during the Jewish month of *Elul* which falls around August and September. In this way we prepare ourselves to stand in front of G-d and ask forgiveness for our wrongdoings. We then ask G-d to wipe clean the slate, leaving a blank page with which to formulate, write and carry out the words of our heart.

We don't need to wait until *Elul* to begin the process of self- reflection.

Practical application might involve regular study, perhaps exploring one chapter of this book at a time with a *chavruta*, a study partner, or in a group led by a rabbi.

Surrender

Ending with the loftiest of yogic goals, *isvarapranidhana* is the fifth and final *niyama*, surrendering to G-d.

The ability to practice a physical surrender in a pose may lead a spiritual seeker closer to mental mastery.

Often, I tell my students to practice in the yoga studio what does not come easily in the world off the mat.

For example, if I am able to release my muscles in a pose, in essence surrendering my will to work the pose, and instead just be in the pose, I will then be able to practice release while at my desk.

We begin with the physical as a more accessible point of focus. Then we move deeper in the yoga class to releasing our mind's grip on the past or the future.

"I am so mad at myself for yelling at my kids this morning."

"I have so much to do later today…how will I get everything done?"

These fluctuations of the mind bring our ego into our practice and prevent us from being in the moment. With continued practice, we learn to quiet these fluctuations by surrendering to the present.

Though the thought of surrender evokes images of weakness or defeat, in reality just the opposite occurs. If I squeeze my hand into a fist, my knuckles turn white. If I release my grip, the blood flow returns.

Moving from a physical practice to a place of quiet in one's mind prepares the student for a deeper path, a path of purpose and connection to something greater than ourselves.

The challenge in Judaism lies in preparing ourselves for the ultimate goals of experiencing the Oneness of G-d and knowing G-d's will.

Commitment to daily prayer with contemplation of Whom we are standing before gives us the structure for such a task.

But how often do we arrive at the *Amidah*, a prayer made while standing before G-d, and realize after half the prayer has been said that our mind's focus is not at all on what our lips are reciting?

The Kabbalists, scholars who focused on the deepest, most esoteric teachings of Judaism, were said to meditate for one hour before prayer in order to have the proper *kavanah*, or intention, needed to speak with G-d.

Recently, a resurgence of Jewish meditation has entered the realm of Jewish practice in a wide variety of flavors. Entering into a meditation practice can greatly heighten a Jew's ability to pray with *kavanah*. However, it is difficult to sit long enough to meditate if one is uncomfortable physically. A physical yoga program or exercise may be necessary to prepare the body for inner reflection.

For those who feel drawn to a blend of prayer, study and action, *Chassidus* may be a path to explore.

The Ba'al Shem Tov, a mystical rabbi of the 18th

century considered the founder of Hasidic Judaism and its body of teachings about the mystical aspects of the Torah, inspired Jews to serve G-d with joy. Divine service is achieved through prayer, *chesed*, acts of loving kindness, and a study of the deeper reflections of Torah.

Chassidus, in Shimona Tzukernik's words, teaches the heart to think and the mind to feel.

If soulful living is the goal, Jews can dive deeply into the depths of Torah to find all that they seek.

The Talmud states that parents are required, among other things, to teach their children to swim. Some of us did not learn from our parents how to swim safely through the sea of Jewish thought. The allure of Eastern philosophy is understandable with yoga studios right around the corner, inviting all to relax, renew, and float in *savasana*.

Jews have been treading water for years, keeping our faith afloat. Perhaps we need to teach ourselves to swim by returning to the familiar waters shared by our matriarchs and patriarchs.

14: Asana, Pranayama and Pratyahara

We began our discussion of the eight limbs of yoga with the *yamas* and *niyamas*. Let us now explore the remaining limbs of yoga.

Physical Poses

William Doran's "Eight Limbs of Yoga" quotes Patanjali's life-affirming description of the gift of *asana*, yoga's physical poses and its third limb:

> "This down-to-earth, flesh-and-bones practice is simply one of the most direct and expedient ways to meet yourself...
> This limb of yoga practice reattaches us to our body. In reattaching ourselves to our

bodies we reattach ourselves
to the responsibility of living a
life guided by the undeniable
wisdom of our body."

Doran also references B. K. S. Iyengar's view that in addressing the body, we access the Divine inside ourselves.

Though I have brought to the surface many aspects of yoga that were problematic for my Jewish soul, I have no argument with Iyengar's interpretation of *asana*. Judaism, like yoga, commands us to care for our bodies and find the Godly within.

Breathing

The fourth limb of yoga, *pranayama*, refers to extension of the breath, or lifeforce.

Students new to yoga are often amazed to discover the tool of breath regulation. We carry this tool with us at all times and most of us are unaware of its power.

A multitude of breath exercises are used to regulate mood.

For example, lengthening the inhale can have an energizing effect. Combined with a heart-opening pose, breath and *asana* can then be used as an adjunct in the treatment of depression. Conversely, discovering the space at the end of the exhale and cultivating comfort in this breath practice can induce calm.

More advanced practices include *nadi sodhana,*

or alternate nostril breathing, *kabhabalabahti* or fire breath, and *viloma* breathing, an interrupted breathing technique.

With the guidance of an experienced practitioner and practice, students can cope with their own mood disturbances.

Amy Weintraub, director of the LifeForce Yoga Healing Institute and author of *Yoga for Depression*, trains yoga professionals to use breathwork and other yogic tools in helping students cope with depression and anxiety. Her ongoing research on the effects of yoga on mood has been recognized and used in hospitals and treatment centers throughout the world.

As a graduate of her training, I utilize her life-saving tools in my classes and private sessions on a regular basis and have seen profound results with just a few sessions of LifeForce yoga. Often, giving someone a breath exercise to focus on allows them a "time-out" from the noise of judgment, fear or worry.

Lifeforce in Judaism is referred to as *chai*. The sanctity of life is valued above all, down to the last second of life. One is not permitted to judge the quality of another's life, even in circumstances of suffering. However, one is permitted to relieve pain at the end of life, without hastening death.

In this vein, extending breath is extending life. In our liturgy, the prayer *Elokai Neshama* acknowledges our living soul that is formed by the breath of G-d.

The translation is as follows:

"My G-d, the soul You placed
within me is pure. You created
it, You formed it, You breathed it
into me, and You guard it while
it is within me. One day You will
take it from me, and restore it to
me in the time to come. As long
as the soul is within me, I will
thank You, HaShem my G-d and
G-d of my ancestors, Master of all
works, Lord of all souls. Blessed
are You, HaShem, who restores
souls to lifeless bodies."

I think of breath as a bridge between the physical
and spiritual. If I can practice awareness of my breath
and exercise my ability to engage in breath, I am
receiving the gift of life. Moreover, I can feel G-d's
presence manifested in my breath.

Internal Focus

The fifth limb of yoga, *pratyahara*, invites the
student to withdraw from the noise of life, to control
one's senses by turning attention to the intrinsic.

Meditation serves this purpose, but many steps
are often needed before one can achieve the quieting
of the mind. *Pratyahara* acts as one of those steps,
following *asana* and *pranayama*.

If I am sitting at the dinner table and the
dishes are displayed in front of me, I may have the
inclination to eat more food, not because I am still
hungry, but because I am tempted by the sight and

smell of the delicious delights. If I remove the food from the table and tuck it into the refrigerator for the night, I have reduced temptation.

On the mat, we dim the senses by sitting quietly, closing our eyes, and turning off our phones.

I am continuously grateful for the tools of yoga practice in life off the mat. Drawing from the discipline of *pratyahara*, my mind softens enough to notice the present moment. Detaching from noxious people, places or things is possible. One is then able to focus on what is truly important, whether it's a loved one needing an ear or a beautiful symphony begging to be heard and felt.

This limb of yoga can be quite useful in so many realms of Jewish life.

Communal Prayer

One custom in prayer is to stand in front of a wall in order to reduce distraction and narrow one's focus toward G-d. In traditional orthodox *shuls*, men and women sit separately during prayer to minimize distraction. I recall my initial reaction to this seating arrangement. Let's just say I was quite appalled by the segregation. I have now come to value my own space while praying. I am in the sanctuary to converse with my Creator, not my husband.

Communal prayer can be a powerful experience particularly when the proper intent and respect is given to the service and those participating. Unfortunately, due to human nature, many people have difficulty dimming their senses in order to focus on what is present. Socializing during the service is not only disrespectful to those who are trying their best to focus on their prayers, but the chatter disrupts the giving and receiving of blessings between congregants and G-d.

My struggle to exercise non-judgment to those incessantly talking and my need to grasp holy sparks during communal prayer is an ongoing battle. Perhaps, I tell myself, the talkers have never tasted the sweetness of quiet contemplation.

Silence is offered on the menu of many yoga retreats.

Some workshops impose such silence and others allow the student to choose periods of quiet by pinning a message of silence on his or her garment. Entering into my first silent weekend retreat, our teachers sensed the panic that was about to set in. We babbled in unison, trying in desperation to get out our last words before evening set.

Our wise and trusted teacher then held a bowl up in the air filled with liquid. As she tipped it, the liquid spilled out onto the yoga studio floor. "Talking too much empties your bowl," she remarked with such profundity. We were there to rest and renew.

At the bell, we closed our mouths and descended onto our own individual islands. Our task? To explore the territory of our mind, without the intrusion of visitors such as friends, pleasure books, or entertainment. Instead, we could take walks, meditate, journal, pray, or if necessary, read books pertaining to self-growth.

After two days on Island Shelly, I had become a local humming the jingle, "Don't worry, be happy."

I couldn't help but wonder how many of our illnesses, both mental and physical, could be prevented by more of this island medicine called silence. Harmful side effects? None that come to mind.

15: Dharana, Dhyana and Samadhi

The sixth and seventh limbs of yoga often become intermingled.

Single-Minded Focus

Dharana, a single point of focus, occurs when we choose to concentrate on one thought or object, while every other distraction fades.

In technological terms, it's analogous to locating a house on an online map. Let's say we want to vacation in Bora Bora and decide to check out the location of a home we plan to rent. Our online map begins with the world view, searches for islands in French Polynesia, and shrinks its focus to the main town of Faanui. Before you know it, we're peering into the living room of a charming rental home perched on a lane lined with palm trees, on the west coast of Faanui. And all the other streets, towns, cities and countries have faded into cyberspace.

Meditation

Dhyana, or meditation, follows. Having arrived, we're no longer gazing at Bora Bora from afar, we are experiencing Bora Bora.

After we have felt the warm island breeze, tasted the fresh shavings of coconut in the just-made pina colada, and heard the strum of the Tahitian ukulele, we settle into the chaise and gaze out into the turquoise water. Our heartbeat drops a notch and we linger in a long exhale. With calm mind and body, we enter into a blissful state of nonthinking, or meditation.

We no longer need to focus on one object, word, or image. We are inside. If we transcend even this moment of bliss to an interconnectedness with all that is, we may feel the awe of being with the Divine.

Oneness

The yogis call this eighth and final limb *samadhi.*

Jews call it Oneness.

Because Judaism is a religion that emphasizes action, achieving such states is not the ultimate goal. Reentry into community is necessary in order to serve G-d.

Therefore, it is important to evaluate the effect

that meditation has on one's connection to others and to G-d, through prayer, *mitzvot*, and repair of the world.

The real work is not in quieting the mind. It is taking the gift of a quiet mind and applying it to human interaction.

Am I a good listener?

Can I practice silence when I really want to yell?

Do I give my full attention to a sacred ceremony without the desire to check my email messages on my phone?

Have I cultivated the patience to explore a text and discuss its intricacies with my *chavruta*, my study partner?

The limbs of *raja* yoga provide a path to move from distraction to clarity.

Judaism provides its own tree of life, abundant with succulent fruit from which we can draw nourishment.

16: Chakras

My father likes to remind me of the recitals I performed in our family living room as a young girl.

After selecting a pink ruffled tutu from our dress-up box, I would twirl, cartwheel, and dance for anyone who was willing to watch. Dance became an integral part of my extracurricular activities and continued with Israeli folk dance as a young adult.

My first husband did not share my enthusiasm for groovin' to Earth, Wind and Fire and I found myself stifling my impulse to dance at the drop of a song. Fortunately, my children were willing partners and our kitchen became the disco floor for many a dance.

Following my divorce, I was in need of some R&R. The Kripalu Center for Yoga and Health was offering a training in DansKinetics, or "dancing through the *chakras.*" This program had my name written all over it.

During my three-week training, we picked apart each chakra, romancing each movement, emotion, location and color associated with these wheels of energy in the body.

We journeyed from the intellectual into the kinesthetic, first learning the *chakra*, then experiencing its characteristics, and then expressing its nature through dance.

Though many of us showed up to become teachers of this yoga in motion, we received the gift of personal exploration. By delving into each *chakra*, we struck emotional chords that had been buried.

The first *chakra*, *muladara*, contains the attributes of safety and groundedness. While rolling around on the floor to earthy, drumming sounds, we assessed our reaction to such movements.

In the second *chakra*, *swadistana*, the sounds of sensual Sade lulled us into flowing watery undulations. The firmness of the first *chakra* was tempered by the yielding of the second *chakra*.

When we reached the fifth *chakra*, *visshuda*, circle dancing erupted, engaging a sense of community.

Sixth *chakra* energy, *ajna*, took the form of a prayer dance that allowed individual expression in one's own space.

Dancing one's prayers resonated a great deal with me. After all, didn't Miriam the prophetess dance with her *chevra* (group) of women, after crossing the Red

Sea?

Dance has been a way for Jewish women to thank G-d and express joy to their Creator for centuries. But I don't think they had *chakras* on their mind.

Floating home from the nirvanic retreat of Kripalu, I plunged into work, leading YogaDance programs to any group willing to gyrate.

After such focused study, the *chakras* had become embedded in my brain like the memorized multiplication tables of grade school. Such knowledge became applicable during private yoga therapy sessions, when words were just not enough to express how clients felt in the deepest parts of their souls.

Through movements, we were able to let the body speak in a language that does not lie. Those feeling powerless had struggles with third *chakra* movements. Women with intimacy issues expressed awkwardness in the second *chakra*.

My career as a YogaDance teacher blossomed, and soon the Jewish community beckoned. Sisterhood groups, synagogue socials, and *Rosh Chodesh* celebrations of the new moon livened up their events with this unique fusion of energy, passion, and calm.

Chakras fit in quite nicely with an ecumenical crowd, but awakening *swadistana* in a Jewish crowd felt like serving shrimp at a *bar mitzvah*.

Music choices were the first to undergo scrutiny.

Barry White was fired, Moshav Band hired.

And my search for a Jewish counterpart to *chakras* began.

The *sefirot*, or emanations of G-d's attributes, have been compared to the *chakras* by many authors.

I wanted so much to connect the dots and neatly replace each *chakra* with a *sefirot*. How convenient and uncomplicated that would be.

But as I tried harder and harder to match them up and get an A on my *chakra-sefirot* exam, I kept coming up with an incomplete. The *sefirot* were not the *chakras*, and any attempt at linking them together felt like cheating.

I would have to take the long, hard route and study the *sefirot* until they moved in and took up residence in my *chakra*-overloaded brain.

17: Sefirot

In YogaDance as I first learned it, we explored our *chakras* to expand our openness to the Divine.

These days, if I were to lead YogaDance in a Jewish setting, I would garb my soul not in *chakras*, but in the garments befitting such an occasion.

The garment of speech would be words of Torah. The intention of the experience would involve the *parsha* (Torah excerpt) of the week or perhaps a theme of renewal in celebration of *Rosh Chodesh*, the first day of each Jewish month. Other intentions might include focus on a particular *chag* (Jewish holiday), or the prayer of opening up our vessels.

The garment of thought begins with my inner focus on the *sefirot*, the ten attributes of the Divine.

And the garment of action would involve the

movements corresponding to each *sefirah*.

Thoughts of the *sefirah chesed* would lead the dancer to expansive, flowing movements, in contrast with the linear, strengthening motions of *gevurah*.

Netzach, or victory, might find the dancer in the center of a circle in celebration of freedom and joy, while *hod*, representing humility, leads the participants to a quiet, introspective space.

As I discussed in the last chapter, a yoga student may study the essence of each *chakra*, wheel of energy, in the physical and emotional body in order to achieve more balance, clarity, or openness.

Identifying one's weakness or imbalance in the *chakra* system can lead a student to work on strengthening a particular *chakra's* energy. Ultimately balancing the emotions in the body will lead the student to higher realms of consciousness.

Evolving Jews may desire greater insight into their emotional makeup and how their weaknesses and strengths manifest themselves. Examining the *sefirot* alive in one's physical world addresses the sefirot in the *nefesh behema*, the animal soul.

Below is a physical representation of the *sefirot* in the human body:

The Sefirot

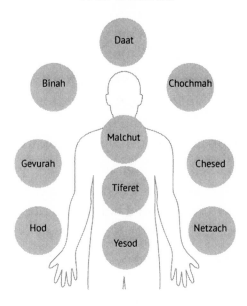

Progressing from our place in the material world, we may ascend to the spiritual sphere, or *nefesh elokit*. Judaism does not separate the effects of our actions in this world from the world to come. What we do, think, and say affects our soul greatly, and prepares it for the world to come. Because our soul is eternal, we must guard and nurture it always.

As part of my journey into the world of unfamiliar *mitzvot*, or commandments, I volunteered for several new *chesed* jobs. I served as a *mikvah* attendant and as a member of the *chevra kadisha* team which prepares the body of the deceased for the world to come.

As a *mikvah* attendant, I assist women in fulfilling the *mitzvah* of *taharat hamishpacha*, or family purity. My role is to observe them in the waters to ensure that the immersion is kosher.

As a member of the *chevra kadisha* team, I and four other women prepare a woman's body for burial by bathing, immersing the body in water, and dressing the body in a shroud, or burial garment.

Both rituals involve recitation of Hebrew prayers, sanctity and modesty of the human body, and a silent environment disturbed only by the necessary instructions.

On one particular evening I was assigned to both *mitzvot* concurrently. While isolated in the quiet, unadorned preparation room, my colleagues and I gently and respectfully poured warm water over the deceased to bring her soul into a state of purity.

Within the walls of this hushed space, my hands carried out the motion of the *taharah*, purifying the body while my soul quivered as if the deceased were communicating a whisper of thanks.

In this most unexpected of places, I experienced comfort in learning this beautiful sacred ritual, gratitude in belonging to a faith that honors the deceased and protects its soul as it departs from the earthly world, and reassurance that I, too, will be cared for when I die. In the care of the lifeless body, I had no doubt of the continuity of this woman's soul into the next world.

Leaving that nameless room, I felt an unspoken yet palpable connection to the other members of the team. Some were my closest friends, others I barely knew.

Leaving the funeral home, I raced home to shower, change and make my way to another *mikvah*, that which prepares a Jew to carry life.

As I watched the women lower themselves into the holy waters, embraced by G-d's presence, I too was held by the beauty of this ritual. I held a towel over my eyes to ensure the modesty and respect of the young women exiting the waters. Words of Hebrew once again were chanted, asking G-d to purify the spirit of the ones immersing.

The mundane in my world had departed that evening.

I was blessed to touch the holy in the crossroads between death and life.

We are all receivers in life. Often a student turns to yoga to receive its gifts. The *sefirot* can be looked at as gifts from G-d. G-d imbues in us these attributes and we in turn give back and thank G-d by expanding our understanding of the *sefirot* and practicing their principles in our everyday lives.

A brief journey through the sefirot follows. For deeper exploration, Rabbi David Dubov, *Kabbalah* lecturer and Director of the Chabad of South London, eloquently expounds on this subject in his article "Sefirot" on Chabad.org, extracting the gems that bring us closer to G-d and to the purpose of our creation.

Chesed

Chesed denotes the emotion of love for G-d and our wish to draw closer to G-d. We express this attribute through acts of kindness. *Chesed* is associated with the right arm and its color is white. The colors indicate the amount of light that is let in. The more light an object has, the closer it is to the Divine. The right arm is used before the left arm in many Jewish rituals in order to sensitize ourselves to being kinder.

Gevurah

 Also called *din*, meaning judgment, *gevurah* represents fear of G-d. *Gevurah* corresponds to the left arm and its color is red.

Gevurah balances *chesed*, as without the boundary of judgment, love would become unharnessed, creating dangerous social situations.

When we are in awe of our Creator, thus containing a healthy fear, we are able to resist the evil inclination, called the *yetzer hara*. Many Jews create fences around dangerous temptations to protect themselves from sinning. For example, an observant man might avoid socializing with a woman in a private space such as his home if others are not present. To the outsider this might appear unnecessary or even ludicrous.

If we as Jews can respect this man's desire to guard against dangerous behaviors we may be better able to see the fence as a source of comfort for him. We might even support him in his quest to elevate the garments of his soul and see the Godliness in his behavior.

Tiferet

Tiferet, translated as "beauty" or "glory," is accessed through our desire to express joy in our service to G-d. Beautifying sacred symbols elevates ritual if it is carried out with the intention of praising G-d. *Tiferet* unites the other nine *sefirot* in the center of the body. This *sefirah* is born from the union of *chesed* and *gevurah* and when in balance, the universe is at peace. The color associated with *tiferet* is purple.

My husband and I travel often, occasionally finding ourselves in obscure locations for *Shabbos*. We pack a "portable *mishkan*," or sanctuary—an extra bag filled with candlesticks, spice box, a disposable tablecloth, and handwoven challah cover.

I become giddy with delight when I have successfully transformed a hotel ottoman into a lovely *Shabbat* table adorned with our ritual objects, Columbia sweatshirts and sneakers tucked away into a bedside drawer.

As if I were Mary Poppins with a bottomless purse, I pull out a *Shabbat* dress, still fresh with the scent of fabric softener. We welcome the Sabbath with newness, beauty and joy.

Netzach and Hod

Netzach and *hod*, located in the right and left foot respectively, are counterparts to each other. We see their location in the feet because it is the feet that take us to a place of action.

Chesed and *gevurah*, in the hands, are the *sefirot*

where action takes place. *Netzach* and *hod* represent earthly involvement. Specifically, we as humans are to ascertain how to implement G-d's will.

Netzach, or victory, represents leadership and victory through obstacles. G-d may present harsh circumstances to us, but we are to see G-d's grace through the difficulties. *Hod*, or splendor, involves the receiving of G-d's message.

At times it is quite difficult to understand G-d's messages because in our world, often the wicked seem to be rewarded. We must acknowledge our limited ability to fully understand G-d's essence, and yet we attempt to move beyond our understanding and trust in G-d's powers.

Hod allows us to replace fear with trust, control with surrender, "I" with "Thou." With *hod*, I can embrace *netzach*, knowing that I am not alone in my battles.

I talked a pretty good talk when I spoke of writing a book. In truth, even I was tired of hearing myself speak of this ethereal goal. The thick notebook of writing snippets stared up at me in the brown wooden to-do box conveniently placed on the top of my desk.

At least it still remained in full view, I reassured myself.

Then one day while teaching a boot camp at the local park, my foot turned sideways while running up and down a set of stairs.

"It's a very common injury, the fifth metatarsal break," squeaked the shiny young orthopedist.

For whom, I wondered? A 51-year-old woman trying to defy the aging process?

Sure enough, the waiting room was filled with baby boomers like me, sporting casts, crutches, and Ace wraps. For the next seven weeks, I was confined to crutches, a rolling scooter, and wheelchair.

The gift? A cleared schedule with which to sit and write. My job was to see G-d's hand in this unexpected accident and welcome the opportunity to finally finish my book.

This was *netzach* at work.

Yesod

Yesod, translated as "foundation," represents the union of *tiferet*, signifying divine male energy, with divine female energy, *malchut*.

Its location is in the genitals, specifically the phallus and uterus. The color associated with *yesod* is orange. Abraham, the first patriarch, was the first Jew to be circumcised, according to G-d's instruction:

> "And G-d spoke to Abraham saying: this is my covenant which you shall keep between Me and you and thy seed after you—every male child among you shall be circumcised."

This ritual obligates us to preserve our covenant with G-d made 3,500 years ago. In essence we are procreating not just Jewish children, but also preserving the foundation of Jewish spiritual and physical existence.

Malchut

Translated as "kingdom," *malchut* represents what is actually occurring in our everyday life.

As Chana Weisberg explains in her article "Malchut and the Feminine,"

> "[Chesed, gevurah, and tiferet] bring the ideas into one's heart where contemplation of the ideas occurs, and...netzach, hod, and yesod...involve acting on one's plan. Once we reach Malchus, our implemented plan now exists in the world. What is significant here is the emphasis on action. Just as the shechinah descends on a home that takes in the observance of the Sabbath (often referred to as Shabbos Malka; the Sabbath Queen) so to the shechinah descends and showers its Godly presence on our dwelling places when we act in a Godly way, through the action of mitzvot."

Chochmah, Binah, & Daat

The above seven *sefirot* represent emotional attributes. The remaining three *sefirot*—*chochmah*, *binah* and *daat*—form the acronym for *Chabad*, the largest Hasidic movement in the world, and reflect intellectual faculties.

Chochmah, wisdom, reflects the first moment of inspiration implanted within our mind by our Creator. If we break apart this word we find *koach*, meaning "potential," and *ma*, translated as "what is." Found on the right side of the brain, its color is blue.

Binah, lying next to *chochmah* on the left side of the brain, takes the seed of *chochmah* and places it in its womb, thus forming a conscious thought. *Binah* is referred to as understanding, and takes on the color of green.

Daat, or knowledge, results from the union of the seed of *chochmah* and the conscious knowledge of *binah*.

With this knowledge we begin to form our character traits, or *middot*. Without the development of this knowledge, we will be misguided in our quest for clarity and closeness with our Creator.

As Rabbi Tzvi Freeman, author of books on Jewish mysticism and spirituality, explains in his article "Da'at: The Knowing I," when children enter the state of *bar mitzvah* or *bat mitzvah*, they have reached the age where they realize the freedom of their existence. Their teenagers' world is turned upside down with the onset of hormones, changing body image, and curiosity about their place in the world. With both trepidation and elation, they begin to ponder their place in the world: who they might want to become and what their options are in behavior and thought.

It saddens me to no end that this time period marks the conclusion of Jewish study for so many young Jews, just as such potential for exploration of purpose and engagement in the world is emerging.

Without continued *daat* in the home and in the school, we are asking our children to find other sources of wisdom that may greatly conflict with the foundation given to us in the Torah.

How does one then balance, without roots in the ground of our faith?

In his book *Letters to a Buddhist Jew,* Rabbi Akiva Tatz addresses an adult Jew who turned to Buddhism because he was unable to find the spark, connection, and wisdom in Judaism that he longed for.

In one of his beautifully articulated responses to Buddhist Jew David Gottlieb's many questions, Rabbi Tatz cites lack of proper Jewish education and learning of biblical Hebrew as among the causes of self-imposed exile of the Western Jew to other religions.

As he says, "In a foreign culture, we are children of the West, not of Torah, and we see the world through the eyes of our host culture. We see Torah through those eyes, too, and that is what makes it inaccessible to us." He explains that Torah lives in its ancient language. Without understanding the roots of the words written by the Almighty, we will not hear what is asked of us and will quickly abandon our obligations as Jews.

This elementary glimpse of the *sefirot* does not begin to uncover the depth of wisdom and light contained in its study. For the Jewish yogi in search of intellectual, emotional, physical and spiritual growth, one may just find the sapphire in the sefirot.

Achieving balance in our everyday lives is a daunting task.

Just when we think we have mastered tree pose, our next challenging balancing pose awaits us. Some days we think we are on top of the world; other days we can barely balance on one foot.

Examining the attributes of the *sefirot* in our own makeup can clarify areas of our lives that need a bit of strengthening or softening.

Becoming aware, then, of our imbalances, we can use tools such as study, prayer, meditation, and *mitzvot* that are deeply rooted in our faith.

As we say in yoga, "ground yourself to grow upward."

18: Aleinu

It is fitting in the last chapter of this book to discuss the *Aleinu*, the Jewish prayer rooted in the earliest days of our existence and found at the conclusion of every Jewish service.

Today the *Aleinu* is proclaimed by Jews of all major denominations. This prayer was instilled into the daily service during medieval times to emphasize the Oneness of G-d and the hope that He will obliterate idolatry from our world. In turn, Jews will then be able to resist adopting the beliefs of other nations living in their midst.

In the first paragraph of the *Aleinu*, we thank G-d for not making us like the nations of the world or placing us like the families of the earth. This liturgy has caused discord in many Jewish circles. I myself have been bothered by our apparent audacity in wishing to nullify the prayers of other "families of the earth."

It is necessary to delve a bit into its meaning before making rash judgments. The backdrop of this prayer is the desert, where Jews wandered in isolation. Christianity had not yet been born. Other than Judaism, no other major monotheistic religions existed; there was only idol worship.

This verse of the *Aleinu*, which stated that "they worship vanity and emptiness and pray to a god who cannot save," was removed from Jewish prayer to minimize Christian outrage and anti-Semitism.

Idols such as cell phones, alcohol and gambling addictions, violence, adultery and more threaten our connection to what is holy and sacred.

Aleinu begins with the letter *Ayin* and ends with the letter *dalet*. Those two letters spell the Hebrew word *ād* which means "witness." We as Jews were witness to G-d's presence at Mount Sinai thousands of years ago. When we bow to our Maker in the *Aleinu* we are proclaiming G-d as the King of Kings, the Holy One. We are praising G-d, thanking G-d, and asking G-d to remove idolatry from the world.

Aleinu is not just rote recitation when we happen to show up at our synagogue of choice. It reaffirms our duty to witness and praise our Creator by proclaiming G-d's Oneness.

Rabbi Eliyahu Eliezer Dessler in his writing *Strive for Truth* explains duty as an obligation one carries out without expecting anything in return. In our world today, many of us want freedom from obligations:

"You only live once; do what you like."

Or perhaps, "I've reached the age where I can do what I want."

The more we desire to remove the yoke of G-d's commandments, the more we distance ourselves from our connection to our Source. Once we move further away from spiritual endeavors that nourish our Jewish soul, we find ourselves in a material world. While we all enjoy material acquisitions, once acquired they remain outside of us.

In yoga, we move from having to being. We enter into a pose and explore its form, shape, and feel. We do not become the pose. Rather, we extrapolate the virtues of the pose: empowerment, relaxation, even revelation.

In the first paragraph of the *Aleinu*, we recite,

> "You are to know this day and
> take to your heart that Hashem
> is the only G-d. In heaven above
> and on the earth below, there is
> none other."

According to Rabbi Dessler, "knowing this day" refers to intellectual knowing and "taking to your heart" creates permanence in one's inner self.

The vehicle for creating a state of connection with our Creator is Torah learning. We may begin the process by acquiring knowledge, but until we perform commandments simply for the sake of love for G-d, no strings attached, our study will remain solely in the realm of the intellect.

Aleinu, therefore, moves us from the material, me-centered world to a place of surrender to the One and Only, our G-d. In this space of surrender where we move from having to being, we are then able to attach ourselves to G-d.

In Judaism we call this *devekut*. Yoga calls it *samadhi*.

One may ask, "Why should I work so hard to surrender to my Creator if I am not receiving some gift or pleasure in return?"

But pleasure is not the goal of the lofty-minded.

Watch new parents with their babies. They're really, truly, present. You know, counting the toes, watching their little lips move, smelling the sweetness of their skin, marveling at the contours of their folds.

No material gifts have been exchanged, and yet the parents are willing to give everything to their babies: love, attention, nurturing for a lifetime.

Children grow up, take their parents for granted at times, and forget to call. Parents long to connect, worry about their children, and wonder how they're doing. A parent's heart hurts sometimes.

Closeness is desired—with parent and child, with the Jews and G-d.

19: Your Soul's Journey

Now what?

Taking in new information and new ideas can feel overwhelming.

In our workshop "Turning Points," my colleague Lucinda Kirk and I provide tools for participants to navigate transitions and actualize their goals.

At the end of every workshop, we ask the students to sit quietly and reflect on their experience, allowing a gem to surface. Then Lucinda asks the participants to formulate a "small win"— a first step in the direction of their desired goals.

As I end all of my private sessions, I am asking you now to do the same:

Sit in a quiet place where no one can interrupt

you.

Close your eyes.

Find your breath.

Ask a question.

"What message did I receive from the reading of this book?"

You may want to reject some of its contents or question its validity. Or you might be inspired to dig deeper and ask more questions.

Is there a gem that emerges?

Before the phone is turned back on, or dinner is made, take a few minutes to sit and absorb, to ponder, to feel.

Then take the next step in the journey of your soul.

Suggested Small Wins

1. Greet your day with *Modeh Ani* before placing your feet on the floor. If you already do recite *Modeh Ani*, try to say it with more *kavanah*, gratitude and intention for your day.

2. Post the prayer *Asher Yatzar* outside your bathroom and read it in the morning after using the bathroom. Appreciate the workings of your body.

3. Engage your heart in a prayer of thanks before eating your breakfast.

4. Talk to G-d in the morning, recalling the

blessings of the past 24 hours.

5. Include an hour of service to others in your week without the expectation of thanks or reward.

6. Light candles on Friday before sundown, for yourself, your family and for the world. Imagine that the light you create is shared with those you love and those you have yet to love.

7. When you find yourself waiting—in traffic, at the doctor's office, in the car pool—find the gift in that space of time to breathe, reflect, observe.

8. Attend a class on Judaism or listen to a lecture online. Torahcafe.com and Aish.com are two excellent sites for learning more about our faith.

9. Find out when your Jewish birthday is and honor the day by giving blessings to others, learning Torah, celebrating the day with friends, or all of the above!

10. Take one small step toward a *mitzvah* that seems unobtainable. For example, if the kosher laws seem daunting, begin with one small step. Perhaps you can buy meat that is both kosher and ethically raised, like the Grow and Behold brand of meat and chicken.

11. Experience a Sabbath meal with another family; if you do not know anyone who celebrates Shabbat, contact your local

Chabad Center or synagogue and ask for an invitation. Don't be shy.

As you explore your own spiritual path, I welcome your insights and thoughts. Feel free to email me with questions or comments to *shellydembe@gmail.com.*

20: Conclusion

Every year on *Simchat Torah* Jews celebrate the conclusion of the yearly reading of our Torah with joyful dance.

I have a particular fondness for this holiday as it marks the anniversary of my engagement to my husband. This day contained both the end of a long search for my *basherte*, my soulmate, and the beginning of a new life together.

So too on *Simchat Torah* we merge endings with beginnings as we read both the last *parsha* and the first *parsha* of our Torah.

In essence, our reading of the Torah is circular in nature.

We are never finished with its study. Just when we think we understand the text and we have arrived at the answer, life changes, we evolve, and the answer no longer fits.

This book is about the evolving Jew and throughout I have tried to encourage readers to examine their ever-changing garments of thought, speech and action. Through my own stories, my intent has been to widen the circle, making room for all Jews to enter and dance.

Why do Jews customarily dance in a circle? In a circle, all are equal.

On *Simchat Torah*, we take turns dancing with the Torah. The delineations of learned and illiterate, Reform and Orthodox, fade. A unified tribe remains, in swirling garments of different colors, filled with sparks of joy, a choir of voices, all rejoicing in the newness of our ancient Torah that is alive today.

May we all dare to wrestle with the obstacles that stand in our path, be it the deities in the yoga studio or the thoughts that muddle our meditation.

May these meditations serve not our ego, not false gods, but our one and only Creator.

Yoga strives to bring the student to a place of comfort. Judaism does not claim comfort as a goal.

Abraham, our first patriarch, knew well the struggle of conformity. He smashed the idols of his time, introducing monotheism to the world.

May we use the strength and wisdom of the Torah to wrestle the idols of today.

The circle is open; shall we dance?

Glossary

A

Ajna: The sixth chakra located at the third eye representing the conscience.

Ahimsa: non-violence.

Aleinu: A Jewish prayer said at the conclusion of the service. Translated as "it is our duty to praise G-d."

Amidah: Also called the Shemonah Esreh, this is the central prayer in Judaism. It contains the three main elements of prayer: praise, request, and thanks. It is recited while standing before G-d.

Aparigraha: non-attachment, releasing the desire to take more than one needs.

Asana: A physical yoga pose or series of poses.

Asher Yatzar: "Who has formed." A blessing recited by Jews after using the bathroom in order to thank G-d for the ability to excrete and keep one's vessels open.

Ashram: A dwelling place for study, contemplation, or practice of Hindu philosophy.

Ashrei: "Happy." This prayer is primarily a Psalm that is recited three times daily. It emphasizes the concept that G-d gives us everything that we need.

Ashtanga yoga: A style of yoga founded by K. Pattabhi Jois. This vigorous practice involves a prescribed set of postures all linked together with breath, creating heat and energy in the body.

Asteya: Non-stealing.

Avodah: "Work" or "service." Usually refers to the work one does in serving G-d.

Avodah zorah: Idol worship (literally, "strange service").

B

Banda: Body lock; involves contraction of the perineum, abdomen and/or throat

Basherte: One's divinely inspired soulmate.

Bar mitzvah: Son of the Commandment. Refers to a boy who has come of age in the sense of being fully obligated to fulfill Jewish law.

Bat mitzvah: Daughter of the Commandment. Refers to a girl who has come of age in the sense of being fully obligated to fulfill Jewish law.

Beit Din: Rabbinic court.

Bhakti yoga: The path of devotion.

Binah: The second intellectual sefirah, "understanding."

Brachmacharya: Control of the senses. Often used when referring to celibacy as a spiritual practice.

C

Chabad: Acronym for chochmah (wisdom), binah (understanding), daat (knowledge). The popular name of the Lubavitch Hasidic movement.

Chaggim: Jewish holidays. "Chag" is the singular form of the word.

Chai: Life. In Hebrew, numbers are represented by letters; therefore every word has a numeric value. The value of chai is 18. As a result the number 18, life, has positive associations.

Chakras: Translated as "wheels" of energy aligned in the body from the crown of the head to the base of the coccyx. Found in Hindu and Buddhist philosophy, these centers are said to keep the physical, spiritual, and emotional body in balance.

Chassidus: The teachings of Jewish mysticism as expressed by the Hasidic sect of Judaism.

Chesed: Loving-kindness. One of the ten sefirah.

Cheshbon hanefesh: Accounting of the soul. A practice that Jews undertake to examine their defects and move toward refining their characters.

Chevra: a group.

Chevra kadisha: "Holy society." A body of Jews who prepare the dead for burial in a respectful, holy way.

Chavruta: Study partner in Torah.

Chochmah: Wisdom, one of the sefirot.

Cholent: A stew customarily eaten for lunch on Shabbat. Since no cooking can be done on Shabbat, cholent must begin cooking on Friday afternoon.

Chukkim: Laws for which there is no obvious rationale.

D

Daat: Knowledge.

Davens: Prays.

Devekut: A clinging to G-d.

Dharana: Single pointed focus.

Din: another word for "gevurah," one of the sefirot.

Dhyana: the state of meditation.

E

Elokai Neshama: A prayer that describes and thanks G-d for the creation, maintenance and destiny of the soul.

Elul: a Jewish month which falls around August and September.

Emunah: the belief in G-d's constant presence in our lives.

F

Farbrengen: Yiddish for a joyous gathering. Often a celebratory event with music and dancing, at which Torah is discussed.

G

Gevurah: The sefirah of strength.

H

Halacha: Jewish scriptural laws that include keeping kosher, observing the Sabbath, and following the laws of family purity and the mikvah. Adjective: halachic, pertaining to law.

Hashem: Literally, "The Name." Names of G-d are holy, and their use is avoided whenever possible. Often substituted for the name of G-d.

Hatha yoga: the physical practice of yoga to stretch, strengthen, and relax the body.

Hod: Humility as we acknowledge the splendor of G-d.

I

Isvarapranidhana: the fifth niyama, which means surrendering to G-d.

J

Jnana yoga: Yoga path of knowledge.

K

Kabbalah: the mystical teachings of the Torah.

Kabhabalabhati: "Breath of fire."

Karma yoga: service to others.

Kashrut: The degree to which food is kosher.

Kavanah: Focused attention on prayer.

Kiddush: The blessing made to bless Shabbat. One Kiddush is said on Friday night, one at lunch on Saturday. The word also refers to a lunch or snack served at a synagogue after the public recitation of the Kiddush blessing.

Klipot: forces which block the light of G-d from our surroundings and our minds.

Kosha: Sheath, used in yogic philosophy to represent a human being's physical, mental, and spiritual layers.

Kvell: To express happy pride, as for the wonderful actions of one's children.

L

Lashon hora: "Evil tongue." Refers to a broad range of prohibited speech, including but not limited to slander and gossip.

M

Magen tzedek: the application of ethical standards for treatment of workers, animals and the environment.

Malchut: The sefirah of kingship.

Mensch: an honorable person.

Mezuzah: Doorpost. The Torah requires certain verses of Torah be written on the doorposts of the house. To fulfill this obligation, a carefully written parchment scroll containing these verses is rolled up and protected in a tubular container affixed to the doorpost.

Middot: Character values; ethics.

Mikvah: Ritual bath, used by women in fulfillment of the laws of family purity, by men before Shabbat and holidays, and by all for immersion of newly acquired cooking vessels.

Mishkan: The "Tent of Meeting" that the Jews carried with them in the Sinai desert.

Mishpatim: Laws which relate to non-ritual matters.

Mitzvah: Commandment.

Mitzvot: Plural of mitzvah. There are 613 mitzvot in the Torah. These mitzvot are the underpinnings of all Jewish law.

Mizmor L'David: The first words, and therefore name, of the 23rd Psalm.

Modeh Ani: "I thank." The first words of the prayer a Jew says upon awakening, before arising, thanking Hashem for restoring the soul after sleep.

Mussar: The improvement of one's character.

N

Nadi sodhana: the yogic practice of alternate nostril breathing.

Nali: A tubular vessel of the body. This is a practice of rolling the abdomen to achieve various health benefits.

Namaskar: to bow or to adore.

Namaste: A common salutation in Hindi, a language spoken predominantly by Hindus.

Naaseh v'nishmah: Means that we first act in accordance with G-d's word, and then can understand the meaning and purpose of those actions.

Nefesh behema: Plural of nefesh habehamit.

Nefesh habehamit: Animal soul.

Nefesh elokit: A person's G-dly soul, as opposed to their nefesh habehamit.

Netzach: The sefirah of victory or eternity.

Niggun (plural: niggunim): Tune.

Nishmat: a Sabbath prayer.

Niyama: Restraints or observances.

O

Olam Haba: the world to come.

Om: A sound believed to be sacred in Hindu philosophy.

Oseh Shalom: "He who makes peace."

P

Parnasah: Sustenance or livelihood. Refers either to a person's profession, or the income itself.

Parsha: an excerpt from the Torah.

Pikuach nefesh: The saving of life. Pikuach nefesh overrides nearly all of the rest of Jewish law.

Pranayama: the yogic practice of controlled breathing.

Pratyahara: Withdrawl of the senses, preparing one for meditation.

R

Raja yoga: The branch of yoga that focuses on calming the minds fluctuations.

Rosh Chodesh: the Jewish celebration of the new moon.

S

Sauca: the first niyama, meaning purity or cleanliness.

Samadhi: A state of consciousness in which the mind is absorbed completely into a state of meditation.

Santosa: Contentment.

Satya: the second yama in raja yoga, meaning to speak the truth.

Savasana: "Corpse pose." In yoga, a posture of complete relaxation.

Sefirot: The ten forces of creation that mediate between G-d and the physical world.

Seva: Service to others.

Shabbat: The Sabbath. The celebration and guarding of the sanctity of Shabbat is one of the mainstays of Jewish life. It has been said that over the centuries, not only did the Jews keep Shabbat, but Shabbat kept the Jews.

Shabbos: Yiddish for Shabbat.

Shalom: Peace. Appears frequently in prayer and psalm, and is often used as a greeting.

Shechina: The feminine aspect of G-d; the presence of G-d.

Shehita: Ritual slaughter. Only certain species of animal may be eaten, and then only if they are slaughtered in a precisely defined, humane way and inspected to be free of disease.

Shema: "Hear." The first word, and therefore commonly used name, for the central affirmation of Jewish faith, said every morning and evening.

Shemonah Esrei: Literally, "18." The ancient set of prayers said morning, afternoon, and evening daily, with some modifications for Shabbat and certain celebrations. There are now 19 prayers in the Shemonah Esrei. The nineteenth prayer was added near the beginning of the Common Era.

Shluchim: those who spread the teachings of Hasidic Judaism.

Shiur: A lecture on a Torah topic. Also, the minimum measure (of food or other things) required to perform a mitzvah.

Shomer negiah: "Observant of touch." A practice of restricting physical contact with a member of the opposite sex in various situations.

Shul: Yiddish word for synagogue.

Siddur: Prayerbook.

Simcha: Joy, or a joyous occasion.

Simchat Torah: "Rejoicing of the Torah." Marks the end of the annual cycle of reading the Torah. The end of the Torah is read publicly, followed by the beginning.

Smachot: the plural of simcha.

Surya namaskar: Also known as sun salutation, this is a series of yoga postures done in a prescribed sequence.

Sutra: Rules that expound the yogic teachings of ethics, postures, and way of life.

Svadhyaya: self-study.

Swadistana: The second chakra, associated with the genitals.

T

Tahara: "Purification." Refers to the respectful washing and dressing of a body in preparation for burial.

Taharat hamishpacha: "Family purity." The laws of marital separation during, and purification after, menstruation.

Tantra yoga: The branch of yoga that addresses ritual, specifically sacred sexuality.

Tapas: The inner fire that creates discipline to control one's impulses.

Tchotchkes: Knick-knacks.

Tehillim: Psalms.

Tiferet: The sefirah of beauty.

Tikkun olam: "Repair of the world." The obligation to improve the world and the human condition.

Tzedakah: "Justice." Used to refer to acts of charity.

U

Ujayi: Also called the ocean breath, the breath is lengthened by tightening the throat and engaging the diaphragm.

Viduy: the Jewish confessional to G-d on Yom Kippur, when Jews strike their chests for sins committed personally or collectively.

Viloma: the yogic technique of interrupted breathing.

Viniyoga: A style of yoga particularly adapted to the unique needs and interests of the individual student.

Virabadrasana: the Sanskrit name for the warrior yoga pose.

Visshudha: The fifth chakra found in the throat.

Y

Yama: Ethical rule for living according to Hindu philosophy.

Yeshiva: "Sitting." A traditional form of Jewish school in which books of Torah, primarily the Talmud, are studied by pairs of students under the guidance of a Rabbi.

Yesod: The sefirah of foundation.

Yetzer hara: The innate inclination to do evil.

Yetzer tov: The innate inclination to do good.

Yirat Hashem: Awe of G-d.

Yom Kippur: the Jewish Day of Atonement, the holiest day of the year.

Z

Zafu: A round cushion most commonly used for sitting on during meditation.

Reading List

In addition to the vast array of historical and religious texts found in both Judaism and Hinduism, the following books and articles provided rich insights throughout my journey. Full publication details are not included because these titles are easily found online and in local libraries, bookstores and Judaica stores.

Books

Asanas: 608 Yoga Poses, Dharma Mittra.

Cheshbon ha-Nefesh, Menachem Mendel Levin.

Jewish Meditation: A Practical Guide, Aryeh Kaplan.

Letters to a Buddhist Jew, David Gottlieb and Akiva Tatz.

Strive for Truth, Eliyahu Eliezer Dessler.

The Vanishing American Jew: In Search of Jewish Identity for the Next Century, Alan Dershowitz.

The Writing Life, Annie Dillard.

Yoga for Depression: A Compassionate Guide to Relieve Suffering Through Yoga, Amy Weintraub.

Articles

"The Additional Shabbat Soul," Rafael Moshe Luria, translated by Simcha Benyosef, www.chabad.org.

"The Branches of Yoga," Mara Carrico, www.yogajournal.com.

"Da'at: The Knowing I," Tzvi Freeman, www.chabad. org.

"The Eight Limbs, The Core of Yoga," William Doran, www.expressionsofspirit.com.

"Malchut and the Feminine," Chana Weisberg, www. askmoses.com.

"OM: Its Purpose and Meaning," Jane (Janani) Cleary, www.theosophical.org.

"Sefirot," Nissan David Dubov, www.chabad.org.

Index

CPSIA information can be obtained at www.ICGtesting.com
Printed in the USA
BVOW07s1856201113

336824BV00001B/5/P